HOBBY TRUMPS HEARTACHE

A Long Hard Journey to Manhood and Old Age

The Memoir of Mike Mullan

PAT CLISHAM

outskirts
press

Outskirts Press, Inc.
http://www.outskirtspress.com

Paperback ISBN: 978-1-9772-1478-2

Outskirts Press and the "OP" logo are trademarks belonging to Outskirts Press, Inc.

PRINTED IN THE UNITED STATES OF AMERICA

To all the good and loving people I have loved or failed or both; especially my two sons, Pat and Ryan, who grew to be the special husbands and dads and men I failed at being early on in life. This artistic work has been inspired from a distance by your virtues.

If you really want to hear about it, the first thing you'll probably want to know is where I was born, and what my lousy childhood was like, and how my parents were occupied and all before they had me, and all that David Copperfield kind of crap, but I don't feel like going into it, if you want to know the truth.

Holden Caufield
The Catcher in the Rye
J.D. Salinger

YOU DON'T KNOW anything about me[1] , but I can tell you, but only this one time. I don't even know why I'm telling you this story, but I do, but it is so unlike me. Other than my small Scriba, NY family, I have only talked openly to 3 or 4 women I've known all my life. Truth of it is, I don't like men much. I don't really have much need to talk to other people either, other than a polite, "Hello" or "How ya doin". That's my world. That's the way I like it. Simple suits me just fine. Anyway, I'm just a plain guy who minds my own business. And I like it that way. I love talking about myself, but I've never met anyone who really wanted to listen longer than 2 minutes at a time until last month. I had been sort of testing the sincerity of this retired therapist neighbor of mine.

---

1   Inspired by Mark Twain, "The Adventures of Huckleberry Finn."

I had a great time with a psychiatrist once a while back. He was doing a Study in which I was a group subject. I got free talk therapy and a medicine out of it. I did love it, especially the free part and the talkin. Tickled myself for making that deal. So other than him and other than the few ladies I mentioned who remain in contact with me, mum's my world.

So this beach neighbor and I have chatted a few times about this or that lately. I don't know what it is but I love talking to the guy. He actually makes me feel like I am somebody, even if I am not. So it surprises the hell out of me, and it doesn't, that I took the time to tell him all that I did. He tells me that I'm an interesting kind of person. Yeah, right! However, he's got the time, I've got the time, and there's this thing about him which really makes me feel good, too. Like a piece of life or the slice of a relationship I've never lived or wanted or needed. "Takes too much focus", I've told myself; "Too complicated". I need simple. So I will tell you the story he got out of me, much of which I had buried a long time ago. Some of which I am proud and some which makes my eyes moist, and I don't really like going there. Most of all, if my story can help others somehow, that'll make me feel good, too. I have never thought of doing something for a group of others before. Too complicated. I just need to take care of me.

It began with my dad's dad who was a typical Irish Catholic Joe lunch bucket in Lowell, Massachusetts. My own dad was born Charles Mullan. I was born Michael Charles Mullan. I never met my granddad, Patrick Mullan. I guess I could say my dad hardly did either or maybe he did. This granddad had 14 or 15 kids and didn't even own a farm! When my dad was seven years old his mom died, suddenly. Little wonder that my granddad, unable to find another woman right away to take on 14 or fewer kids, dropped off my seven year old dad and his younger siblings at the local orphanage. Period.

You know, granddad Mullan had to work to take care of all those kids so he couldn't be running a household. I mean by then, some of my dad's siblings were already married so they took in the older kids who could mow lawns and do chores and take care of themselves. The rest of the younger kids had to go into the orphanage. My father and the younger kids ended up in the orphanage, except that every Sunday, my granddad visited that orphanage to see every one of his kids. He brought them each a penny, every Sunday of his life. Other than that it did not last long, since he died when my own dad was 11. Period.

As was often the case, several years later, my dad's older sister, Joan, reunited him by taking him in with her family and kids in Syracuse. While the younger kids stayed in the orphanage, my dad began his years in Syracuse at about 11 in his sister's home with her welcoming husband, with 4 nephews and nieces a couple years younger than him. No natural parents, no other siblings to count on, and no home to go back to, nowhere.

I go by Mike and I don't know whether Charles is my confirmation name or baptismal name or nothing about that. I don't know where I got it. I was born November 23, 1942. Somebody said just after the War started but I don't know. I wasn't around that soon. I don't keep track of those things. The proud parents of this newborn were Charlie Mullan and Mary Mullan, Mary Davis Mullan. So you can put for the record that this is and was a really Irish family. I used to think my granddad Mullan came over straight from Ireland but then some people told me that it was really his parents who were born in Ireland. So I don't know for sure. Of course I never met that set of grandparents because they were both dead by the time my father was 11. So my dad was actually born in 1916 or 1917. I'll say '17. Now my mom was born in 1917 too but she wasn't a Lowell, Massachusetts girl.

I'll tell you how it was. She was probably born in Oswego, New York, right on Lake Ontario. How they met is sort of a long story but I'm gonna tell you anyway. My father was taken in, like I said, by his older sister, Joan, who had moved to Syracuse from Lowell. She had married a longhaul trucker, a good man, hard worker. They saw that my dad got to school and such. As for my mom, her mother married my grandfather Davis in Oswego, NY. They had two daughters, one being my mom, Mary, and Rita. At some point that marriage fell apart. All I know is what my grandmother Leger Davis used to say.

"There's only one reason for divorce."

That was infidelity.

"So we had to set it up."

Nothing ever happened that way so a friend of hers came and sat on the end of the bed. They recorded it and took a picture of it. Went to the Court. It was agreeable by both parties. Both my grandparents wanted to be divorced but they had to create the circumstances which fit the legal laws of that era. So then my grandmother moved to Syracuse with her two daughters. So just like my dad, my mother was already there with her one sister, Rita, where they went to school in Syracuse, public school. I can't think of the name of it. So this is my sense of humor. My father was probably looking for some action and you know, maybe that's how they met. I really don't know.

Now, as far as school for my parents, I think my dad probably went to the seventh, maybe the eighth grade. And my mom, I never really asked her, but definitely went to high school. I don't know if she finished but she told me about this gal she used to pal around with so I know she attended high school. They both had divorced parents so they sorta had that in common. That was sorta hard in Syracuse in those days. Being divorced was definitely not the norm back then in Syracuse. Then later, I don't know when, when her kids were grown, my grandmother moved back into my grandfather's nice big old farm house. Nevertheless, her role was that of his housekeeper and cook kind of thing. She slept upstairs and he slept downstairs. And most weekends, he went off to Syracuse where he had social connections. They got along just fine. No tension.

My parents went and also had two kids. They had two boys, me and Martin, my older brother. He was born six years before I was born. You gotta calculate that. I don't do that kind of math. I mean, I can do math calculations but I just can't get that one right now. You know, it was like the late thirties. I can do them in my head. I'll do it for you.

'42, '40, '36. He was born in 1936. So he was Martin Mullan. We had this 6 year age difference so we grew up sorta separately. But as far as sleeping arrangements, I guess we really did grow up separately.

See, this is another kind of odd thing about my family. My mother's parents had a meat market in Oswego where my mom and dad worked for them, H B Davis Market. So my father worked for my grandfather Davis and my mother worked in the store as she had growing up until the divorce. And at the time my parents married, they were in Syracuse where they actually bought a house. So when they began their married life in Syracuse, my grandmother didn't think that my mom was doing a very good job of taking care of the first child, Marty, so she saw after him a lot, I guess. So she was the live-in housekeeper and cook and volunteered to do child care for Marty.

After all my parents were quite young when they had their first child so my grandmother took care of my brother a lot. Then when they had me, I guess things weren't going too well. They had the house in Syracuse so they moved nearer to Oswego because that's where my father worked in the meat market for my mom's dad. And my mom worked there because, you know, when you have a family business, that's what you have to do. Everybody has to work.

So our family resettled in Oswego with my father working at the meat market with my mother. But rather than us being a family of 4, and I don't know how this happened, but my grandmother, remember, had became the housekeeper for my grandfather, her ex-husband, in their big local Oswego home. And I don't know how this happened but I think they concurred on the fact that my brother was better off with them. There was no fight or anything. Since I was a tot, I don't know how it went down but my brother always lived with my grandparents. He never lived with us in our house in my memory.

Now, we only lived a mile apart and my mother and my grand-mother cooked many a dinner on a Sunday, mostly for our 2 families. We had a lot of interaction, you know, like we weren't cut off and not speaking to each other. Marty just grew up with our grandparents for his parents and I grew up alone with my parents. Two brothers separated from one another, but not really, because we didn't think anything was really different, ever, to this day. I mean, I really have to giggle at that because I felt we really had a close knit family but my brother grew up with them and I grew up with my parents. So today, I mean, it seems sort of weird to say, but back then, everything was great. Am I kidding myself about close to feel good? Every Saturday morning Marty calls me on the dot at 730am and we chat. I really am proud of him for that. I don't know if we are close though. Part of me feels close and part of me feels on another planet. Of course I exaggerate. I suppose I should take a minute and make a small correction and that is, we all lived actually in Scriba. And that's right outside of Oswego. If you leave Oswego and go north to Mexico, New York or New Haven, New York - a lot of people don't know those places - you take Route 104 from Oswego east to Mexico. I say that to a lot of people trying to describe Scriba but when you leave the city of Oswego, you then go into Scriba. And it is a real town because I had to pay my taxes there but you're not going to find it on the map.

I probably shouldn't say this but I'm going to anyway. My mother and father got married because my mother was pregnant so whatever year that was in school, that's what happened. Marty was born in June 1936 so I figure they got married in 1935, which makes them both 18. As far as the religious influence in our home, my dad seemed to like the Catholic religion, whereas my mom was born and raised Baptist or Methodist, one of those lefthanders. And I would say that as far as who took the lead in teaching me my prayers and stuff like that, I would say it was pretty even, though without a doubt, I was closer to my mother. I sided with her for the longest time, privately of course, because of the way my father treated her sometimes when they would have these terrible, terrible shouting matches.

You see, my father, what I was gonna tell you about my brother's birth is this. Until my father died in 1977, nobody knew about, and nobody talked about, that early pregnancy. Nobody ever knew that. I mean, some people knew it but they kept it quiet. Us children didn't know that. When my father died suddenly in 1977 right down in our basement, my brother was working far away. I was working for the Union Hall on construction, digging ditches my grandmother used to say though what I really did was push a broom. Marty made it back, of course, for the funeral. That's a long story you don't need to hear. Marty was on a business trip. It was Christmas time. It was the 22nd of December I think. On construction you have to be there. The construction is organized out of the Union Hall. So as soon as the funeral is over, I tell my brother I got to go to work. I had a job then. And so I told him, you sort out the stuff that is important from my dad's little office that he had there and all, and I will get it to the attorney. My mother is somewhere in the house. I am gone working. My brother is alone sorting. He comes across the marriage certificate. He looks at it and he says to her,

"The date, it's torn off. There's no date."

And that's when my mother confided to him about how they got married and how he was born early. So their anniversary was always one year off. They moved their anniversary back to coincide with my brother's early delivery.

You see, this gets even more complicated, because apparently, at some time after I was born, my mother cheated on my father and he caught her. And so with my parents when there was tension, I guess my father had his own tensions. My father would go . . . he would . . . he was a binge drinker. He'd take off for three or four days, maybe a week I guess. I guess the week was the longest but usually three or four days on a binge. He'd return when somebody went to pick him up or he ran out of money. But he would call her a whore or when things were tough, you know how men are, bulls or bears, he was louder than her. She was smaller than him. So I just didn't think he was treating her very good every time they had one of those episodes. They really shook me up because they both yelled so loud and angry that I was sure every time they were going to kill each other. Makes me shudder even now as I flash back to it.

When my mom was dying, as I was taking care of her by myself, she told me this affair part of the story. In the last week or two of her life, with no one else in the room but her and me, that's when she told me that story about the affair. She even told me the man's name. I'd say it but I don't think it would make any difference. I knew him. So I was really pretty shocked about all this for certain. And then this missing piece of the fighting history gave my father a lot of leeway, in my brain. But, too late, he's gone.

Now, if we go back to the very beginning like my earliest memory, for me that's probably – of course I remember going to kindergarten. It was in a two room country school house in Scriba. My class had four to six students. And there were 8 grades in the whole school. The year I was there they added on the kindergarten because, well my father had enough influence that it had kindergarten the year I was due. And then they eliminated the kindergarten. Now I am not saying that is true. That's only my belief. There were four grades in each room and that year there had to be an extra grade because of the fact that they added a kindergarten but they only did it one year.

Now I don't remember how they taught all these different grades at the same time. But I do remember, all the classes were the same size. I mean, eight would be big because we had 10 or 12 chairs and we would go up front. You know, the little ones, not the fullsize ones. And we would go up and set in those chairs, and the teacher would teach us. And when we were not sitting on those chairs, then we were sitting at our desk where we had something we were supposed to be working on, I guess, while she was teaching another segment up front. They did it! That's all I can tell you. I don't have a clue how anybody could teach that way. So rather than just going there for all 8 grades, they changed it and separated off somewhere near the junior high 7th and 8th grades. So I went there for all six grades.

Because I am old now, as I look back, I know I really liked arithmetic but the rest of it, I was just a chubby little kid. We had our own business you know, food store. My father was on the heavy side to some degree, and my mother used to take a lot of diet pills to try to control the whole thing. At any rate, I don't have a lot of fond memories back then. I was a fat kid and if they played baseball, I was the last one picked. Someone had to have me. And I didn't do well at it so school was really hard for me, really hard. We would have to stand up and read aloud. "Dick and Jane" was almost a . . . I'd have to say this looking back on it. At the time it did not seem like anything traumatic to me. But as I look back on it, I think, I just stumbled through the Reader, "Dick and Jane", the best I could. Pick a word here and there and kind of get by. I am going to tell you the truth. It is just something I really don't care to dwell on because, I guess, being almost 20 years old when I got out of high school, it's not something that turned me on very much.

When I left my 6 year elementary educational career behind under my dad's Scriba town influence, I was able to fail the seventh grade very easily in Oswego. I don't know how they did it back then; all I know is, I did not move along with my friends. I did not participate well. I did not know how to study. I probably didn't do homework. I remember the teacher would call on me in spelling, Mr. Egizi. He would call on you, give you a word, spell it. I didn't have a prayer. I don't know where he got the words from. It wasn't like he gave us 5 or 10 words to study the night before. He just came up with a word. He was the homeroom teacher so his responsibility might have been spelling. I don't know. It's too fuzzy. I don't know that I ever took a class from him. I think he was a science teacher. But in homeroom he must've had other responsibilities because I was forced to spell.

I don't know. I never prepared much at home anyway to be perfectly honest with you. I mean, working in the store really never interfered with anything. It was the reading. The reading! I just never read very well. To this day I feel I don't read very well, not very well at all. I can't say that loud enough or long enough. A woman I dated for a certain period of time told me that the newspaper is written at a fourth grade level. That was a lot of years ago. I don't know whether she was right are not. But I took it to heart and it made me feel a lot better because I could read the newspaper pretty well. And I still enjoy reading the newspaper. I sure do. Here I read what I call the Blade. It's got another name but I can't recall exactly what it is. Not interested in the name.

Now as far as my buddies and friends back in school in those days, first of all when it comes to girlfriends. Not! The Wheeling kids, a couple of them and Johnny Chapman I hung around with; Maury Stein a little bit; the Butler kids. One of the things that drew us together back in those days, after school was out, not many of us had television sets. In fact probably in the first part of that schooling, nobody had them. And the Chapman family got a television set. And I'd say it wasn't very big but we'd be 12 or 15 or 18 people in their living room watching the television set. I don't know what the hell was on it but it was a picture. It was a picture, like in your house! And that was a big deal. Watching a television set? Wow! I only say that because I'm old. Especially in downtown Scriba, we were a little backward so that was a big deal.

Now in high school, if you want to talk about junior and senior prom - they had it; I did not have it. It's hard for me to look back on it and say anything. I can easily say shyness, or still being fat. In other words the ugly girl in class did not pursue me to go to the dance. The same guys I hung out with in junior high went on with me to high school. They might've been a little bit ahead of me or little bit behind me but we all still hung out together.

As I look back trying to think of a hero or a role model I might have had in grammar school or high school, I really can't think of anybody. I liked the cowboys on TV not "Dallas". Roy Rogers and . . . at least Roy Rogers. He was my first hero. Cowboys were fun to watch on the big screen. Some kids were into comic books but I sure wasn't. Again, the reading. No way. There might've been comic books lying around but I don't remember ever picking one up and being interested enough to look at it and read it or page through it. On the other hand I was a cub scout and a boy scout. I made that radio with the string in the empty tin can. I had the full uniform naturally. I learned to do all those things in the Webelos scout handbook like tying knots. I can't do one now but I could get it enough to pass the test back then.

I'll just tell you something about high school. I look back on this as a really interesting moment. A long time ago photographers used to have their own studio in like an office. And out front in the display window, they would have all these beautiful frames with photos in them as samples of their work. So in high school my last name was Mullan. And the girl who sat behind me, Terry Murphy, she used to have her picture in the display window. So as I look back on it in hindsight, with the standard of living that our family had, I pretty much got to do anything I wanted to do. Like nobody ever said about anything,

"We don't have enough money".

In fact my father made a point of that. My father never said that we don't have enough money. He'd tell me,

"We can make this work. Just tell me what you want", and he'll do it. He'll get it done.

So I went to the Oswego Speedway. It opened in 1952. Only 10 years old. I did not get there much at all the very first year. I only made it once and I didn't like all that dirt flying in my face. Then they paved it, and I went. I went to every race there till somewhere in the 70's – 25 or so years, every Saturday night. So I would tell this really pretty girl, just tell her, the one who had her photo in the display window, that I was going to the races; and she said to me once, I'll never forget this:

"I'd love to go to the races."

Too dumb to know it. Too dumb to hear what she was saying. I regret that terribly. She used to have a portfolio of herself. Kept it in her locker or something. And she used to show it to me - without a lot of clothes on sometimes. I would see this picture of her. Remember those long draping things the strippers used to wear? Long time ago. She showed me a picture of herself wrapped in this feather boa. And that's all I could see. The rest of it was skin. And I would say to her something about that and she would say,

"Oh I've got a bathing suit on underneath that."

That's the biggest reason why I went to my 50th class reunion. I wanted to see if she'd be there. I knew her mother. Her mother used to trade in the grocery store that I worked in. I guess I sorta knew pretty much everybody in town. And I would've loved to see if she turned out looking like her mom because her mom look like a raving beauty to me. So she turned out to be a no show at the reunion. I asked around about her. But nobody seemed to have a lead on her. And I am not capable of searching around online to find her. Not capable yet I own a computer – a laptop. I can search for symbols, stock symbols.

So the other really important thing about the Speedway story is that I used to tell my mother, my father and I grew up together - every Saturday night. The two of us were at that Speedway, sitting right next to each other, every week that they ran. On Saturday night everybody knew where the two of us were going to be. We had to get back from somewhere sometimes so we could be there. We're now as far as the refreshments; here's how that went. My father rarely drank. He would have a beer at home occasionally. But when he went to take a little trip, he drank Canadian Club. And my father never drank Canadian Cub any other time. He'd have a beer. Not a big deal. They have a name for people like that - periodic alcoholics. I'll tell you my refreshment ritual later.

Eventually my dad's father-in-law who owned Davis Market backed away from the business, semi-retired, and my dad took it over. And I don't know for sure, but I don't think my dad bought the business from him or leased it. I think my grandfather just said,

"I'm okay so you take it from here".

My grandfather decided he wanted to become a farmer for a little while. Planted a lot of raspberry bushes and bought a tractor; cultivated around everything. And I don't know if this was his early retirement or what. He was just a good startup guy. And raspberry farming can be very lucrative but it's also very high risk, and I think he learned that the hard way.

Now the Market was called a meat market, but in my world, you had enough groceries in there that you could do your regular shopping.

So there was dairy and bread and groceries and dry goods but mainly it was a meat market. Now we didn't have barrels of pickles or barrels of fresh baked rolls. So the only thing I remember open like that is Nabisco. And it came in a cardboard bin that Nabisco either gave you or sold you. I think they probably gave it to you. And it had a door on it. And you opened the door and picked out the Nabisco crackers or cookie type that you wanted. They were not boxed. That's the only special visual kind of packaging that I recall that was unique for that era. They converted rather quickly though to boxing it up and sending it out that way. That self serve option was a little too tempting for too many customers to help themselves to one or two. They were a nice treat for me, I remember, since I worked around it all the time in the store.

I tried to help out wherever I could. I used to go down to the basement because the canned goods were kept in the basement. And I would go down with a box. And I think I probably did it myself but my memory is that somebody would tell me what to get and then I'd bring them upstairs and put them on the shelf and line them up, labels facing out. Somebody asked me how old I was when I started. And here's how it worked. The store was open from six in the morning till 6 o'clock at night. So if I wasn't with my grandmother or my brother in the house where Marty was being raised, I was at the store when I wasn't in school of course.

I must have learned a few things other than just opening boxes and stocking shelves. All I remember . . . I used to put up potatoes. You got potatoes delivered in a 50 pound bag back then. I think I made a peck out of them, that's 15 pounds. And if I went to 16 pounds, my mother would be all upset with me. If I went to 16 pounds, that was just out of the question. Also, you had to put your eggs into one dozen packages back then. They used to come in a crate. So I would move the eggs from the crate to the dozen size packages and try not to break any. It would have been a poor move to break one.

So where my dad was the real professional was with the meat. We didn't buy any precuts. Everything was what they call hanging beef.

Hinds and fronts. Hind quarters and front quarters. He knew exactly how to be the perfect butcher and my granddad probably taught him everything in that regard. We always had an employee there too, one or two. Now as far as who the customers thought ran the store, because we all worked there, I would say it was my father. It was not a very big store. And when he would disappear on those three or four day binges infrequently, my mother would just run it.

So somewhere there in seventh or eighth grade my father closed up the store. It just wasn't doing that well. A&P came to town. The bigger supermarket you had, the better you were. He would have had to buy another building in order to expand and keep up to compete. Now I would like to say that A&P came to my father and said, "We would like you to close and here's $50,000 or $100,000 to go away".

However, that did not happen. I would know. Even though I was young, I like those kind of things so he would have told me for sure. There would be no question that he would have told me. In fact he would've told the world. My father was not at all shy, though there was nobody as shy as I was.

I can't say if my brother is as shy as I am. After all he was raised by a different set of adults or parents. I really don't think I can speak to that. I have a friend who coined the phrase, and now that she's met some of my family, my brother uses it. She has coined the phrase, Mullanisms. My brother worked for the government for all of his career in finance where he went to the top of his ladder. He had a series of very, very important jobs. When he retired, close staff had a little gathering for him. He didn't want them to have anything but I guess, the way it sounded to me, the people right around him did at the time - maybe 10, 15, I don't know, 30, pick a number. His secretary spoke or somebody spoke for a bit and said,

"Mr. Mullan's idea of small talk is,

"Good morning!".

So perhaps he was quiet like my grandfather Davis was, really quiet.

I try to be like my grandfather as best I can at this point in my life. H B Davis was a doer but much more on the quiet side. He and my grandmother, and my parents, just added so much to my making it and getting by. Makes me almost cry that it took me this late in life to realize that and really feel it. In fact I think that my grandfather has served as my most important role model for all of my life, now that I think of it.

He had the business; he owned it. He started it. My grandfather started in retail on a cart with a horse and buggy on the road in downtown Scriba. He used to tell me stories about how he would go to farmers because he had products on there that farmers obviously needed or wanted or whatever the horse and buggy carried. And one morning, my grandfather said, another huckster on the route called out to him,

"Chubb". So the salesman says, "I got this barrel of flour".

So we're not talking about bags of flour; we're talking about the barrel of flour.

"I can give you a good price on it"

So he told him the price of the barrel of flour. So my grandfather says, "Nah, that's a lot of flour. I don't know that I can use a barrel of flour."

So my grandfather pedaled around the countryside. And as he told it to me, as time went on during the day, farmers all had hard cider on hand. And he'd generally say no, and sometimes he'd say yes because he didn't want to offend anybody. And by the time he got to the end of his route that day, feeling no pain, he ran across this flour salesman again.

And he told him, "Hey, I'll take that barrel of flour now".

So I tell you that story as an example of how I felt my grandfather was a normal human being, you know what I mean? He was real quiet and conscientious about his work and everything, but he didn't mind having a few glasses of cider from time to time either which sometimes might have mildly impaired his judgment about buying flour wholesale. So he went from being a horse and buggy peddler to owning his own meat market and grocery store in Oswego with a real nice big home in Scriba. And of course my parents and me had a real nice house in downtown Scriba too.

I stayed with my passion for that Speedway every Saturday night, and I absolutely loved it. So I made sure I got myself a car at 16 years of age. I mean, I always worked for my dad so I always had a paying job as a student. I was very fortunate because in this little town of Scriba, my family was well known, well thought of. The guy who ran the body shop, he was on the main road. And he used to put out - actually he didn't want people laid off from work. So he would buy wrecked cars and those out of work people would fix them up to put them out by the road for sale. So when I got ready to buy a car, he had a '54 Chevy down there that was black, and looked pretty to me. So I stopped down to see him. We struck a deal at, I don't know, probably $495. He allowed me to pay him $50 or a $100, whatever it was back then, a month or whatever number he decided on that I could cope with. And I paid him until the car was paid off. No interest. Ronny Schmidt. I'll never forget him.

At the high school that I went to, the enrollment was probably 1000. And there was about 250 in my 1st year class when I was 16. And I hate to say this but I'm pretty sure that nobody else in that entire high school had their very own car. See my sense of humor is that I could've sold myself a lot better if I had that pick up line gab. But I didn't; that's all I can tell you. And you know what I liked about that '54 Chevy? That it was a car. That's all I cared about - that I had a car. Now you want to know what I didn't like about it? It was a standard shift – a gearshift. And that is the only one I have ever owned in my entire life. And the fundamental objection that I had to it was that, I had to do it. It was just too much trouble. I mean we were buying cars. I think my father had a brand new 1948 Buick – again a stick shift, which makes it sort of sound like he was well-to-do. However the truth is that he just had good friends at the bank.

The way it worked in my world is that in 1956, automatic shift transmissions were available and I was on it. And that was the next car I had. I was a happy buyer. That second car was a '56 Chevy but it wasn't a convertible. I had to wait until 1964 to get one of those. Nobody was into trucks and all that stuff back then. I pretty much always got a four door because they were popular. And you might think that was because I could fit more buddies. Not. Acquaintances were not my strong point and they still are not. I told you the story before about my brother and small talk being a Mullanism. And in the same way, in the grocery business which I used to work in, I felt I had a lot to do. And I wanted to get as much done as I could. So when I saw somebody in the aisle, I would just say "Hi" or "How ya doin", and keep on walking by moving away. I never stopped to engage. The way I looked at it was, I had a lot to do and I was sure I could get it done, yet I wasn't going to get it done by talking. Now maybe back in my school days in the hallways, there was what we called city kids and country kids. And so you sort a hung around yet I wasn't going to get it done by talking.

Now maybe back in my school days in the hallways, there was what we called city kids and country kids. And so you sort a hung around with the group that you grew up with. You might ask, was I a city kid or country kid? You gotta remember way back on I told you, I went to the little country 2 room schoolhouse. We didn't even have water. We didn't even have plumbing. Somebody filled up like a 5 gallon thing, and you go over and get a drink. And then the outhouses were attached to the back of the building on the outside of course. You went to the back of the room toilet door entrance for that stuff. And no paint was wasted on boys or girls signs. First come, first served. Might have only been one stall - no flush. And as far as sanitation goes, there was nothing set up to wash your hands. And to this day, I don't wash my hands. So I'm guessing in the metropolis of downtown Scriba, there was probably no public health department going around educating the public about safe practices. And we didn't have any typhoid and we didn't have any epidemics and so, who knows? And I've managed to survive until today - something I think about all the time, about life.

So back to how blind I was about trying to attract members of the opposite sex. And to my amazement, as I would drive my car, my '54, around town, if there was anybody on the curb or the sidewalk noticing me, I never noticed them. The only thing I remember doing with my '56 is, we used a go to church, that religious education program that we could get out of school early for. Plus you got a half a point on your transcript with that Regents diploma program which New York State had. You had to have 18 points saying you got so many points for whatever you got or whatever you did. So I figured that the religious instruction class would be good for me because I could get another point. And then I could get an impressive Regents diploma and get out of school. With my adversity to testing, after three good years, I didn't go to the test because I didn't like to do them. So I never got the credit. So I only got three quarters of a credit, one for each year and because I lacked that one quarter of a credit, I never got the Regents diploma. After working at it for those three years, it just became water under the bridge. It don't mean nothin anyway. So I used to take people, drive them over to the religion class because I had the car. One of them was a guy named Nelson and he probably brought a couple buddies. Most of the kids that I went to grammar school with were either Protestant or Baptist, whereas I had gone to the Catholic church in Oswego where my father used to go as a member of the parish.

I'm just going to say this and be done with it. In the Fall most high schools have a football team who play on Friday or Saturday. And after the game especially if your school won, there might be some driving around town blowing horns and celebrating. I never went to a high school football game in my four years. I went to absolutely no sporting events connected to my high school. The only extracurricular activity I was part of was, I was on the visual aids where you ran the projector. And I probably got that because that's what my older brother did ahead of me. So the teacher took me right in right away because my brother was the captain of it. The attraction for me was that you didn't have to say anything. You just had to operate the machine. And it wasn't too complicated. I always say this about life. God took good care of me, I hope. Cross my fingers.

My grandmother remained a housekeeper in my school days for

my grandfather. Remember, my brother lived there. My grandmother had another daughter, my Aunt Rita. She had a boy and girl; my mother had two boys. And that was my grandmother's family, you know. She was really good at keeping people together. That's what I call it. Somebody else might call it something else. She did this holiday dinner, all the time, without fail. Around those holiday times, she made sure that people get together. My mother's sister, Rita, lived in a little town called Cape Vincent about 65 or 70 miles away along the Saint Lawrence River - about 1 ½ hours away driving the car. My grandmother never ever got turned down when she got everyone together at holiday time. When the word got out that she was serving dinner, we all showed up for sure. My aunt's husband, a quiet polite Italian fellow, would basically sit through the dinner. Then he'd get up for his routine holiday drive to Syracuse where his own family was celebrating with another dinner. His wife and kids would sit there through the rest of the meal together with us having a great time. I admired that in him.

Now my dad, he didn't go nowhere because he was an orphan so he didn't have any other family to go to. I just talked about that because a married life is something like how I really know nothing about. Although, I am an uncle by my brother having two boys and a girl so I have two nephews and a niece. I have a phone conversation with one of them occasionally. One nephew comes down here to the beach because my brother owns the condo across the street. And I guess he's gonna take it over, the oldest one. And he's going to be the owner of it, I guess. So I see him occasionally because he's down here. And I can say this now with some actuality, about the generations. Unless you have someone who draws the people together, in my opinion, generations seem to separate like sheep from the wolves. I don't know what they call it. I see him a couple times a year. Something I learned about living here on the beach . . . when people come here to visit, if they did not come here to visit you, you're not gonna see them. Because they came here for a reason; they have a purpose. So I have begun to accept that. So I don't really reach out to too many people anymore who come here to visit. I was trying for a while to be like my grandmother, I thought, but since I don't have any kids, I guess that's not the thing to do. I tried to be the gatherer but it didn't work out like I thought it would. So I have accepted that. I would have enjoyed being closer with them but, none of them are really close. And I don't know, I'm just going to say it. The way I look at it is, my grandmother was a unifier. She had at least three siblings, two brothers and a sister. Yet my brother's wife is an only child. I tell myself that maybe her mother may not have been doing gathering the way that our mom's mother was. I'm not saying that's the way it is. That's just the way I think about it. So maybe her children don't get the warm fuzzies. That's how I put it together in my world to understand it or to make sense of it.

When I graduated high school, and it came time for me to figure out what my next step was going to be, I drew a blank. When it comes to me about going to college, it's hard for me to remember or to elaborate. But I would think that in my mind back then, it was a definite no, a big no. Like Ma & Pa Kettle used to say, I didn't do buckle under very good. It's that simple. I did go to a community college for half a semester. I don't believe I made it through the whole year. Like when they got to the midyear, they just told me it was time to move on. And since I was young, I guess I was a little bit crushed, but more relieved, because without a doubt, the academics were hard.

So I had went to work for my father in another grocery store. My father became a store manager for a company called P&C. And I worked for him as a part time person during high school, too. That is how I had money enough to buy cars. So when I graduated high school, I stayed with the part time job, four years. I say that because I don't really know. I did go to work full time when P&C opened another store in the same town which was really rare. My father sold the idea to them, which they had never done before. It was a small company and the president told my father that they only opened new stores by using a watchacallit, a protractor on a map to plot out a fifteen mile radius. And then they used that boundary to identify how much further out they might build a new store. But anyway, they upgraded to a new store and my father went on to be a supervisor of some type in this chain organization. At any rate they built this store, and I went to work full time there, in the new store. I think my father was on the road then with that company as like a Regional Manager.

So at the new store I was a grocery clerk doing all the things that I had been doing for my father in our market during my high school years. And sometimes I would work at the register so I handled money. Then they put me in a training program so I could learn the meat department. You might not like this tidbit but I liked it. Makes me chuckle. They would let me break a front (half) because those were the cheaper grades. I was not allowed to break a hind quarter, where the expensive cuts were, but I could break a front. A half is half a cow. The front leg is in the front and back leg is in the rear. The hind is the whole rear half, the tail. So you can see what I mean by that term front half. So you split the cow in half. And you take the half which has been split, and split that in half down the middle, top to bottom; and one side becomes the front quarter and the other side becomes the hind quarter. Front leg, hind leg. So the more expensive pieces of beef come from the hind quarter. So I never got to break a hind quarter but I got to break a front. Boy, it's a long time ago! There's a rib you pick out; you don't pick it out. It's a rib that you come down with the boning knife, and you slice it as best you can - all the way through the thing. That makes it so you're down to a quarter and you get that done. I think you had to use a saw a little bit for some of it, yet some people could catch them with their hand, but I used to have to catch them with a barrel, and then pick them out of there so they would not hit the floor. So when you get that done, that's like the major thing, you know. And then you take the thing to cut smaller. Butchers generally in my time would do that with a power saw, just like a saw that a carpenter would use except made for food cutting so as to cut the smaller pieces. I even still have all my fingers. God forbid.

Hey, I got in a little trouble with the meat manager when I was doing that training because I'm left handed. By adapting I write right handed because I broke my left arm – still have the scar there. It was a compound fracture. That was a big deal in the fifties, compound fracture, so I learned to write right handed because of that fact, but I eat, the important thing I do is eat, with my left hand. I can use either hand, you know, to some degree. I wouldn't call myself ambidextrous. I could shift, not too hard for me to go from one hand to the other. I used to slip the knife over to my left, and do some stuff over there; and I'd put it back in my right hand. The guy told me that this was risky. You had to use one hand or the other, preferably the right hand because you're less apt to cut somebody than when you're switching hands; or when you're drawing it back somewhere as you're using the other one so I tried to be as politically correct about that as I could be. I never thought about it. Just something I was capable of doing.

I can't say I really like all that butchering exposure and training. It was greasy and your hands were always... God, I don't think anybody wore gloves. I'd have had an apron for sure. I don't know if I had a white long coat or not. I know I had an apron because some blood would run out of things here and there. Something you don't need to know, just because I cherish it about the grocery business. Maybe it's worthy but when you roll a roast, and in my day rolling a roast in my father's - my Davis Market days, you rolled the roast. You had a little special tool you poke through there and you put the string through it. Then you drew it back and then you tied the knot and rolled the roast. Well, when I got to come around, they had a cone like a megaphone that opened up relatively easy. You got that roast together, trimmed it up, whatever you did, kind of flopped it together. Then you shoved it through this cone and the cone had this stuff in there that held it together. Looks like, almost like a nylon stocking, but a lot of holes in it. So anyway, in my world when I was doing that, you had the bag. You put those in the bag. Not everybody did that, but where I was, not that I had anything to do with it, they just told me to do that and I did it. You put that in a plastic bag, that nice rolled roast, and you tied it up at the top or wrapped something around it and then you'd hang it in the walkin cooler. When you got ready to cut that roast up, put it out for sale, it would be - the word was juice. It was blood. The word was juice, in the bottom of that plastic bag. You would take the hamburger meat that you were gonna make hamburger out of. Then you'd puncture that rolled bag over the pan so that all that juice went into that hamburger. The hamburger wasn't ground yet. It was just meat that was gonna be ground. Then when you ground that hamburger, you ground all that juice into the mix. Supposedly it's a weight thing.

I just tell you that because that's part of my real deal. On the other hand, you can not weigh the sheet which absorbs the liquid on any of your package cuts for sale. It's against the law. Can't weigh that. You call that a tear. You have to put a tear on it. You could do it . . . if you did do that and you got caught, you'd be fined. So it was pretty easy to get caught. You know, there was people that would come in and check occasionally, not very often, but if they weighed up a bunch of things and they were off, they would not be warm and fuzzy. They'd fine you. So they pretty . . . everybody's pretty legitimate when I - at least when I was involved in it. So even back then, a government agency was looking out for the customer.

My dad and I both had our military service, unusual as it was. Up our way, all you did during my time which was Viet Nam was join the Guard. We never got called up and it seemed, every one knew we would never get called up so it was safe for all of us who went that route rather than active duty. Personally I never thought about going in the military, you know, for real, on active duty. On the other hand my father was in military service. In fact he was in World War II. But he tells the story about that. He went really late. And he was on his way over on this troop ship when VE Day happened. The war ended.

One of his jokes was, "They heard I was coming".

My mother used to claim, with her Irish sense of humor, that she got him drafted. I don't know if those things are true. They were living in Syracuse at the time so if she did, I don't know how she would've done it because she wasn't connected like she was in Oswego. He didn't have to really go at all because he had kids I guess. Plus he was a re-capper. He did re-caps for Firestone in Syracuse. So he could have had a deferment for young kids and a deferment for working in the rubber industry which was critical for the War. But somehow he got Orders or she saw that he got Orders, and he got on the troop ship to Europe, when they ended it.

Dad had gone to Army basic training somewhere in northern Florida where I took a picture later. He used to display a picture of himself in St. Augustine, FL on a bridge where there's a pair of lions on each end and on each side of the road. The picture was always in my house. My brother and I both went there and got our pictures taken by the way. Mine is gone now though because I had a car stolen here out of the garage a few years ago and my pictures were in the trunk. And they're gone. I don't need them anymore. I consider that a good thing, those pictures. Too much a part of my life. I would like to have them of course. I don't have anybody to pass them on to anyway. My brother's got them and he's got kids so everything's good.

Speaking of Marty, my brother . . . when he got out of our high school, he went to college and took accounting. He got into a sorta new private Jesuit Catholic college called Le Moyne in Syracuse. And the way it worked back then is, Le Moyne didn't have any dormitories. So he stayed with a woman who rented him an upstairs room as a student. And then he would come home during the summer. The interesting part about his living in Syracuse is that I didn't really lose a brother. My mother went to visit him every Sunday, every week, to bring him up a care package. Many times she took me with her. Remember now, I am like sixth or seventh grade when he was a college freshman and that's how we did it. Our mother tells this story. She sent him a dollar every day in the mail during the school year. So in no way was he out of our family life. And of course Syracuse was only an hour away in the '50's because when you live in the Oswego area, you realize that if you want to go to any decent stores, you have to go to Syracuse.

Marty has had a wife forever and ever. After my brother left college, I sorta forget, but it could not have been too long because they have celebrated their 50th, and they're heading toward 60. Now that I go back that far, I was his best man. And that is the one and only wedding that I was ever a best man for. I was in another wedding party just as an other guy. Can't think of what you call that. . .

I stayed with P&C until before my father died in '77. My father went on disability and I had the opportunity to go on construction, because some friends - friends of mine in a sense, but a friend of my father's who knew me, worked part-time in the grocery store until he went on construction. His name was Harold Brown. He was pretty well connected to the Labor Union in Oswego. So I was having a difficult time because I was working nights for that chain grocery. The leadership - the new leadership since my father went on disability - didn't quite see me as like my father did. So they told me when I went on nights, it would just be a while, you know, just kind of get the night crew straightened out so they could . . . back in those days stores weren't open after nine o'clock at night. We only opened Thursday and Fridays until nine o'clock and the other nights, we closed at six. But maybe by that time we were open until nine every night. I think we were open until nine o'clock every night. So we'd go to work at nine or nine-thirty or ten - work until six in the morning. I didn't get along well with working nights, so I tried, and apparently during that time, that's when my father died suddenly. So the time frame of this story is around when, I am pretty sure, I was working those nights.

So I had a job change opportunity but at the same time, the first girlfriend I ever had decided to break up with me at that same juncture - in that same time frame. And I was having a really, really hard time with that. Like I'll just say it. If it's good or bad, you can hold your ears. I was getting laid regularly with her. Pretty much so, right? It was all new to me and it was wonderful Now that I look back on life, I really don't pay a lot of attention to people; see if they're happy or not. I try to make an effort nowadays because it's a pertinent thing to do.

At any rate, she decided . . . I didn't realize about marriage and all that stuff. To me, I just thought she had a good time and she wanted to get married. She didn't make it as clear to me as I thought. I even offered to buy something and live with her, but she wouldn't. She didn't have any interest in doing that. She wanted apparently . . . I don't remember marriage being talked about, but in her mind I guess I'm sure if you talked to her, she'd explain to you that it was . . . You know, at any rate, she broke up with me and I was like lost. Man!

So I went to - my father was dead - I went to my doctor in Oswego, my medical doctor. I told him that I'm just functioning, you know. I go to work. I come home. I go to work, come home, and I don't eat much. I guess I probably lost a lot of weight, you know, so he said that I was depressed.

He said, "I'll give you some Valium to take".

So I said that will be good. Valium was a popular item back in those days. So I took the prescription like I was supposed to and the great thing about it was, I slept really good. I slept most of the time. So I went back to him. I said what I just said, you know. "This is really nice, except all I am doing is working, sleeping and that's pretty much the crux of it." He said I needed to go to see a psychologist.

Well, in Oswego I guess, probably at that time, there wasn't any practicing psychologists maybe. I don't know, but he recommended a guy in Syracuse who was attached to the mental health – a mental health agency in Oswego who was let go. They were probably buddies or something, so he mentioned the guy and said he would be in touch with him and he would be in touch with me or whatever. I went to see the guy. I can't think of his name right now, but he - I thought when I went there, this will be really good because I'll be like going to the medical doctor. I'll go once and it will be over; I'll be done. I kind of liked that, you know. So he started talking to me about coming back and things and I said to him sort of probably almost like this because I knew what the price is. I always asked those things; what's the price. I told him that sounds expensive.

And he said, "How would you like to come for nothing?"

I said, "That's sounds really good."

So he said, "I have a test drug for depression".

I guess I learned over time, it lasted a year, the Study. A year!

So I saw him a few times and the man apparently that was in charge of the work to deal with the test drug would come in and sit sometimes. And I seemed to like him a lot. He seemed a lot nicer to me than the guy I was talking to. Yeah, I probably would have been better off if I'd stayed with the doctor. He might have pushed me some, but nonetheless, I did what I did. So I said to the doctor at some point in time, I said, "Is there any possibility that I could see - I call him Fred?" I don't know what his name was.

"Oh, yeah," he says, "You can do that. That's no problem. That's not a problem for me."

So I started seeing this other - wasn't a psychologist. He was probably a psychologist as opposed to a psychiatrist. And I got along really good with him and he treated me really nice, like I liked to be treated, you know, for free, for free. I know. Only could happen to me. So I got along really well with him. As a matter of fact, he fixed me up with a woman. He had a wife, but he also had a girlfriend on the side. So I got to meet this friend of hers with his girlfriend. Now his girlfriend was really dynamite and mine was like, not very good looking at all, at all. How's that for blatant? So I only ever saw her once and then I saw him again for the Study stuff.

You know, we still got along really well and he . . . it was getting near the end of the time of this program to be over, you know. He said to me at some point in time, he said . . . he made me aware that it was coming. He gave me the - there were always sealed bottles. He gave me the bottle and I'd been tapering off from the drug, because back in those days, I didn't like to depend on the drugs. I got lots of them I'm taking now, but back in those days I didn't want to take nothing. I'd been tapering off.

He gave me the bottle while saying, "That's your last bottle; come back in two weeks".

So I went home and never opened the bottle. I don't think I ever took anything. If I did, I just took some I had left over from the previous thing, you know. I went back. I threw him the bottle with the seal on it and said, "There's your bottle". So I hadn't taken any. And with that, we parted ways very, very friendly.

He said to me, "You know, if you ever need anything, I'll give you my number, you know, my office here and I'll tell them just put me in touch with you, you know, if you want. I'll get back to you right away. If I don't talk to you right away, I'll get back to you right away."

I thought, boy, that's gonna be really nice. I kind of like that.

So I went on my wildly ways, whatever I did, drinking, driving my car, whatever and feel good. And I was in a little place in a tavern; I think it's in Liverpool, but it doesn't make any difference where it is, close to Syracuse, really drunk. And I decided in my infinite wisdom I was gonna call him up. They had a pay phone. He had told me that he had to go in for surgery, something to do with his heart. Not a major operation, but he had to go in for surgery and he'd be in surgery and I knew that time had passed, whatever the surgery time was. So I called up the office and told them who I wanted to talk to and they said I can always - for whatever reason, I knew they were giving me the run around about where he was and what he was doing. I said to them in my infinite wisdom, I said "What's the deal here? He told me I could call up and I - when is he gonna call me back? He said he'd get in touch with me."

She said, "Well, when Fred went in for the operation, he died, on the table."

I said, "Thank you" and hung up. That was the end of my experience with – I didn't need it. I was able to overcome it. I didn't need my hand held again. So hey, truth is stranger than fiction. I thought I needed more support and then since he died, I decided I'd handle it.

Hey, when you're young, you think you are - you're sure you're capable. I did - yeah. I haven't been - I've been back a little bit since I got down here but I was always - I did do a little more counseling somehow through a church thing. I knew I could do that in Oswego but not a lot. And when I came down here to the beach, I did a little bit in the beginning. I haven't done anything for at least fifteen years.

So lemme return to my heartbreak when my girlfriend moved on to pursue others. I am in my mid 30's, and my job is either at the end of the night job at P&C grocery store or at the beginning of my Union job from my Dad's buddy. I had no plan or clue. I was just following an escape from the night job. There again, God, I hope, takes good care of me. Somebody does. As I went on to learn, a Union job, when they're building a nuclear power plant that takes about 5 to 7 years to build, cannot be bid. I never knew that but there's no bid. It's called time and materials. What that means is, so everybody hears this don't understand it. It means whatever you spend, you get your profit over top of that. I don't care what the number is – say 1%. Could be 2%. I don't know what they got. I don't know what anybody got. Doesn't make any difference what you get when the basis is, the more you spend, the more you get. That's 1% of this number; make the number bigger, that's 1% of that number. And they treat you really good.

I'll tell you this story about that and just a little, just a side line. When I first started out, in the winter it was a big deal if you get called in to shovel snow because they had to have paths, you know. Somebody came to work, they had to get out to the site, you know - clear paths. So they called me in. I don't know how big the snow blower was then but we're not talking about paved roads. It's a construction site. You know, there's a pile of dirt here and you know, covered in snow and you just got to pick a direction and use your head and shovel it. If you hit something, you know, with the snow blower, well - but anyway, whatever. So we would have snow by the yard - especially on the shore of Lake Ontario. So they called me in and I knew this going in. I'll just say you went in 6am, might have been 5am. I have no idea. They call you in some ungodly hour! Then you got to work your shift because, you know, you're hired on. So at the end of my first snow shoveling, I told the person that was in charge of calling, not to call me again. "Take my name off that list." Everybody wanted it - overtime. I mean, I am a greedy guy but I know in my own mind, I'm not into inconvenience. So I never did that again.

So my day job was, they started me off to be on the concrete crew. Laborers have the pouring of the concrete, Laborers Union 214. So you have charge of getting the product from the mixer to the form. They got a - it's done by air pressure when you're going up. They push it right through this tube and it goes way up to the top of the form to create a wall. So that was supposed to be a cherry job because all you had to do was get the pipe set up so you could connect the hose. Now that I think about it, it was all pipe and on the end of it, there was a hose that could do that connection. So, I couldn't stand it, could not stand it. It was a lot of work to me. And it was dirty. I was coming from the clean grocery business. So I just said to my friend; he was a Union shop steward on the job. "If they need a carpenter helper, I think I could probably do that." So, with a snap of his fingers, I got transferred.

Most of my career I call myself a carpenter helper. I don't know what they called it, you know, but yeah, I didn't know nothin. Nailing, not a clue. Hammer? Huh? The carpenter had to tell me everything. Yeah. I got so I could - I probably couldn't do it today. I knew the terminology that they wanted when they built the scaffold. It was metal scaffold back then. Grandfathered in the metal workers because the carpenters had that job years ago, so you just toted this metal stuff and they put it up.

Well, I stayed with the Laborers Union as a carpenter helper for the rest of my career. But really, I just did what they asked me to do, as long as it did not inconvenience me. They needed a broom sweeper, I did it. They needed supplies, I get a cart and push it over to them. I was 55 years old when I took a pension from the Union. They were my employer. So their pension to me and my social security were to be my primary sources of income to retire with.

Now I also . . . this was the fun part. I had a job that was my own creation. That is, doesn't make any money. When my mother passed away, she was a hoarder in the fact that she thought she could buy things and then her grandchildren would be able to sell them and make a lot of money. I had a 60foot length of basement by whatever the width was, 24 foot, with lots of trails going around it of all this stuff that my mother - perfume bottles – collected all my life until she died.

This is gonna be a little hard. In my childhood experiences when my father would have his rages, they probably weren't like anything to worry about, but I didn't have any standard for what . . . yeah, so somehow I thought in my brain that me being there would stop anything from happening, which I know wasn't true because the man died alone in the basement so you know, I was there. I was upstairs. I saw him just before he went down there, before he went down to the basement for the last time, with his dog at least. I was working on construction. I didn't treat him very well at that point. I had turned my gloves inside out so they'd dry and all what goes on in the morning. He was trying to help me with that and I remember distinctly saying, "I can get that!". I'd done that a lot of . . . so just telling about these details fills me up kinda.

For whatever reason, one acquaintance of mine who I have in Oswego tells me my mother didn't do me any favors. She doesn't say that derogatorily. She just says it because she was around for a long time in my life and I just stayed there after my father died. It wasn't a lot of years, I don't think, before my mother died, but whatever it was, I stayed there about 13 years. Maybe lack of confidence, you know, too . . . it's interesting - confidence, or whatever I'm talking about here. I've known this girl since she was, I'm gonna say, less than 10 so she still knows me and she's known me. My father and her father were really close friends so she's known me a long time. I think she meant, you know, you could . . . my word, the way I'm gonna word it is, people can take too good a care of you.

Sometime during that 5 – 7 year construction boom, I bought a rental house in Oswego because with this nuclear power plant being built, rentals were just terrific. It was like people would come from .

. . well, we had people staying in a trailer that we rented to them. We had people from Texas. Came from Texas; worked in Scriba because it was money, money, money. So I bought a rental house when I was working in construction, plus there's a college in Oswego that really helps with rental houses. Lots of kids don't want to live on campus so the rental business is always good on the west side of Oswego because kids don't want to live on campus. So mine was on the other side of the river but I didn't have any trouble with it at all. My mom was still alive. I remember she helped me clean up the apartment house when I bought it. She helped me clean it suitable so I could rent it. One unit was rented. It was three units. One unit was rented and the other two was empty. The small one was the one rented which is, I learned, really nice because the guy had been there forever. The two bedroom ones were empty but I needed to clean those up – painting and such. I did the painting and stuff like that. I needed to clean them up. Make sure they were presentable to be rented. No hot water because I wouldn't turn on the hot water. They had individual things for the hot water so they were shut off because there was nobody in them. I wouldn't turn them on so we cleaned. I cleaned, she cleaned, we cleaned with cold water. Wasn't the most smart thing to do probably but that's my world. I can't help that.

I did really well. People were begging me to take and rent these apartments and I . . . I actually paid it off early. I didn't have any debt on it. So when the power plant opened, construction was over and everybody went home. I really failed miserably at the rental business then so I sold it. That's how I come to own a place on the South Carolina beach. I did one of those - it's some kind of real estate tax shelter. You could do a switch. Go from one rental property to another. No capital gains tax. That's how I bought the rentals that I have in this building and still lived in the north, you know, because I had the money put together.

There again I was tunnel vision. When I bought a couple rental condos down south here near my brother's beach condo, I was still living in northern New York State. I had a friend. He told me a condo on the beach was a great magnet to attract women. But I didn't even get it then, and that was 18 - 20 years ago when I was in my middle 50s. That was, I think, when my mother was dead for sure. She died in '90, but I wasn't smart enough to capitalize on his know-how. You know, I had these condo units down here. So he was trying to smarten me up about what normalcy is. And I didn't get it. I bought the units to rent, not to be in the hunt. I wasn't interested in anything else. Just give me a pile of money. That's what I bought them for. The first year I made some money, so much money that I bought a second one - an efficiency that was attached to a two bedroom unit facing the ocean. More on that later. I am getting ahead of myself.

I never intended to live with my parents. Just turned out that way. I never had a plan. Just went from year to year. My girl friend at that time, when we had sex, it was always at her house. I mean, she would come to my house when my parents were there, but never any private activity. I mean, she knew my father. She worked for the P&C. But I would never even think of that, to be honest with you, back then. Having sex in my own bedroom with my parents or mother in the house just never occurred to me, though it still embarrasses me now.

Living with my parents was a fine fit for a guy like me. Never a problem, no matter what I did. We didn't have any arguments. Even after my dad died, my mom of course loved me being there I guess. I'd get drunk, but not troublesome. Not a word from her. I'll tell you a story about that. Just understand how easy . . . how easy she was. She used to make a dish called goulash, which is, I don't know what it is for everybody, but hers was basically just hamburger, macaroni, tomatoes, a little bit of onion but not enough to even talk about that. But as we engaged one another, our relationship got better over time for whatever reason. She had made some of that and I had been out drinking. I got home and it was summertime, real nice weather. I decided in my infinite wisdom I'd have some of that dish, cold out of the refrigerator. And I ate it and it didn't go well so I went outside and threw up. Course, summer time; windows all open. I come back in and fall into bed. My mother's room was on one side and I was on the other side. The door was probably open. And she pipes up with, "There's more goulash in the refrigerator". So how much more understanding could anybody be, you know what I mean? I could tell you other things probably, but that's the best one that I know of. She knew I'd gone outside and thrown up. She could hear me. She was awake. Maybe she was awake all the time when I came in. I have no idea, but she was awake then. It still makes me laugh.

When I would go out to taverns then, I tried to move around some. I didn't do it to socialize. My goal was getting drunk. That's the truth. I look back on it and I'm sure that's what I enjoyed, whiskey and water. From time to time, I became aware of the fact that sometimes I didn't get very much whiskey so I would make it known to the person that they could put a lot of ice cubes in the glass but that is water not whiskey. "So do what you want to do; I'd like to have it taste . . . I'd like to have the effect I want to get." Anyway, I was able to get that message across.

As for my consumption to reach my goal, how many whiskey and waters in an evening would I consume in order to reach the appropriate level of intoxication? I can't tell you exactly, but something I generally did when I drank. No matter where you drink, it's like buying a can of peas or whatever you do. You go to one bar or another. They're basically the same price so I used to always take every swizzle stick and put it in my back pocket. After I bought, that's where it went - my back pocket. And I always figured it balanced out 'cause if somebody happened to buy me a drink, I bought them one. Just a way for me to analyze. What I was really trying to do is see if they screwed with me with money. I'd count my money before I went out and then I could count it when I got up the next morning. I'd count the swizzle sticks and add the price and I could usually come out with . . . generally I was not too bad. I felt pretty comfortable with the whole thing. I never had to return back to the bar being upset about the fact that the number didn't come out really good.

Any rate, the way I'm gonna tell you this, this is the way I'm gonna tell you this. Generally I did that when I got to work in the morning because I had the swizzle sticks so I would count them. Then was when you worked with the carpenters. You had a partner so my partner was by the work box and I was counting my swizzle sticks. I knew what was in my wallet so I was balancing out all right. So he asked me, because he'd seen me doing it, how many I had. It was a teen number. I can't tell you. Could have been 13 or 15, but it wasn't many more than that for sure, but it was a teen number that was in my back pocket. So I did a good job that night is all I can . . . couldn't tell you about every night, but that particular night it was a teen number.

He said, "I can't imagine you being here" is what he said to me.

"They pay me. I got to come." Years of practice.

I don't know what time frame that was in. I certainly didn't drink that way all my life. I never drank two days in a row, ever. I went out to get drunk when I went out. That was . . . I didn't feel my body needed to have that happen to it all the time. I'm not saying I never got drunk two days in a row, but as a general rule, didn't happen two days in a row. Never had a compulsion to do back to back nights. Lady told me that . . . the lady I told you about that my mother didn't do me any favor. I told her that story. She told me I am not a drunk because people . . . drunks don't do that. You know, they don't stop. They just continue on.

I have some people, well, not very many, but there was a little lady in Oswego at the race track. Used to call me, "The drunk". Hey, that's what she called me. She's a friend of mine now. I could call her on the phone right now. Just what she called me back at the time. I used to take a half gallon of vodka and a gallon of orange juice to the Speedway. I used to wrap the vodka up in a blanket because you couldn't take glass in but I would take the orange juice in a plastic container with all the ice cubes and stuff like that. I could steal the cups from a concession stand so I didn't have to buy any cups. So anyway, at the end of the night, the vodka was all gone. I didn't drink it all. I gave some away - anybody wanted to have a drink, you know, but I did my share. At the end of the night the vodka was always gone. There was always orange juice left. And it wasn't a half gallon either. That's the way they do those liquor bottles, you know. Looked like a half gallon but it wasn't a half gallon. I just know I can look at it today and you can look at the bottle. It says something. It don't say 64 ounces, you know, so...

That was a stupid part of me. On the other side of the coin, and to be honest with you, I don't know how I glopped on to this. But I can just tell you something that happened to me when I was younger. I had a friend who opened . . . it wasn't my friend but he opened a barber shop right next to my house in downtown Scriba which was pretty something to have a barber shop right downtown. And he had big old dogs that he trained and hunted with and for whatever reason, I guess I took a liken to him. I have no idea why that is, but his name was Paddy Vagnozzi. His father was obviously Italian and his mother was Irish. He used to go by PV a lot, but anyway, Paddy was, I look back on it, he was a big influence on my life. I was probably still in high school, I guess. I don't know where I was, but I can tell you, I think he bought a - it was in the fifties. Maybe not. It was in the fifties. Wasn't a forty because he had a '49 Packard when he moved out there. That was an old car in them days. So he bought . . . my father was selling cars on the side. They sold Hudson's and General Motors. GMC trucks oddly as it may sound today but that's what they did. He bought a truck from my father because he knew my father. He was living next door, you know. So at any rate, so I was trying to give you the time frame, but any rate, whatever it is. He was interesting to me.

Paddy was a gambler, an investor, an entrepreneur. He was his own boss. There wasn't any situation where . . . he had been a barber before he went in the Service. For whatever reason he didn't pursue that afterwards. I don't know what he did pursue, but he decided in later years he was gonna be a barber again and he got . . . you have to get a license in New York State to be a barber; just can't hang out a shingle so he got his license and opened this place out there. He was open three o'clock in the afternoon until nine at night. He was basically retired probably.

PAT CLISHAM

He wanted to run his dogs during the daylight hours. He wanted to do that; then he could open up for the nighttime, cut hair, maybe make a lot of money.

I don't know if that's true, but that's my life. So he began to talk to me about how he bought some things in this thing called a stock market. I don't even . . . I can't even tell you the conversation. Bottom line is, he got me to buy my first stock for whatever reason and this was the story he told me about a company called National Distillers. I could buy either 10 shares or 20 shares. It was either one of those numbers I was gonna buy for my first small purchase. We decided on that number. He told me I think it was worth about $40 per share. So in 2 weeks or 3 weeks or some hypothetical date out there, if I bought 10 shares, I'd have 20 shares. And if I bought 20 shares, I'd have 40 shares. And in my mind, I thought this is gonna be great. Gonna double my money. Right? And I know now that they announce the split date. I know that now. I'd never known that back then.

But anyway, he took me down to Oswego and we went across the street from the hospital on the front porch of some guy's house who was a stockbroker. I paid him $400 bucks to buy 10 shares of National Distillers. And when it split, I can say for sure that I was disappointed, but apparently not enough disappointed to worry about it. I kept it. I had it for a long time. And he did another thing with Chiquita Bananas. Back in those days, that was a public company, but he knew the banana market enough to know that the banana company would decrease in value. He'd buy it when it was down and he'd sell it in the same year when it was up, and make some money. I never did that. He told me about it. I listened to him.

Somehow that's the only . . . oh, I know, the other thing, I almost left that out. During that time frame I was in high school. And in New York State during that time, you could subscribe to the New York Times. I have to make up a number - $1 a week or $.50 or something. Monday through Friday you get the New York Times in the school. It was a school thing and you didn't get it on the weekend, but you got the New York Times. So I bought the New York Times because my parents had this business that we've talked about. Anytime we ever got away for a couple of days, we had somebody who worked for us or something. We arranged something so the business didn't close and we would go to New York City. I can't remember how we got there. Those things always bother me.

I can remember being there. We would go to shows in New York City, and the Rockettes back in those days, just to date this really a lot. The Rockettes would perform, I think, after you'd seen a dog act jump through the hoop things and some kind of thing went on prior to that, all at Radio City Music Hall. I don't know how much, but at least that I remember. And after that, you would see a movie. Movie! We'd see a movie! We saw those things and then a movie. I thought I died and went to heaven. The room was gorgeous. Anybody that's ever been there has got to know that. I think it's the best I've ever been in. I say rooms. I gush at the theater rooms in New York – wonderful. I try to go to some theater rooms - terrible. At any rate, not a big deal.

Any rate, where was a going? So I sent off for the New York Times. I got it for the reason I thought, when we go to New York City, I'll be right on the top of my game. I can say I want to see this or I want to see that. I want to do this; I can read it, point it out. We can live it at home, you know, when I'm looking at the New York Times.

So I was working for my father in the grocery store, putting product, merchandise, on the shelf. I noticed lots of things sold really, really well. Campbell Soups and Hellmann's Mayonnaise and Heinz Ketchup – Jello. I don't know whether it's been taken over. At the same time a lot of things did not sell very well. I thought, well, just what I thought you know, these things sold really well. For some reason I turned to the financial pages in the New York Times and I saw those companies, Coca Cola, Campbell Soups, General Mills, I think, whatever one of them. Kellogg's, not General Mills. Kellogg's was a big seller. I mentioned Jello because it wasn't called that. It was another company that had been taken over. I knew the company because I put that crap on the shelf. I could read the name of the company. Royal was the competitor, believe it or not. Didn't sell worth a shit. Anyway, so I thought, I know where that time frame is buying the liquor company. I got a feeling that's before - I think I bought the liquor company first. I got a feeling, because I dealt with somebody, God only knows. Over time I've dealt with so many people so many times. I can't even remember because you get with somebody. You had to have a broker and you had to make a transaction.

So I bought some things. Fay's drugstore was a chain that I bought that it turned into Rite Aid so you can tell how long I've been around. They took over Fay's drugstore many, many years ago and now they're about to fold up. But anyway, well, they tried to be absorbed by Walgreens and the government squashed it. I keep track. My sense of humor nobody gets. And they made a lot of money on that. There again, 10 shares, 20 shares, all I could afford to buy. I probably bought it right there from that guy on the porch like I did. Then I bought Kellogg's and Heinz. I bought, I mean, I'm squashing all this together. But you're probably saying, thank God, because I just did, you know; you're talking probably 3 or 4 years, you know.

I bought little things. I actually got like, Disney. I got Coca Cola, too. Kind of had a choice back then. It was real easy. You could just check a box and you could get the certificate if you wanted to – not just a paper statement. They would hold a paper statement for you. It was easy. Basically all you had to do was ask and you got the certificate. They sent it to you so I got the Coca Cola one. I got the Disney one because I wanted to see. I wanted to see them. I was disappointed in some. I think I got the Campbell's one or the Kellogg's one or something and it was like, why did I get this dull certificate. I think a lot of people liked stock certificates. There probably was a time when that was the only way you could do it. They probably just gave it to you, you know. There was probably no paper statement. It was probably your responsibility to hold onto the gd thing. When I came along, it was an option. You can get a certificate or not get a certificate.

So I was truly relatively young when I took up this hobby. Like the New York Times, for sure I got it the first year I got to high school, though I was 16 already. I know I got the New York Times because that was an important thing to me because I wanted to know what was going on in New York City. I was working in the grocery store so I started looking at those things. I looked at it consciously before I ever went to get the New York Times. I mean, I could, I guess if you stock shelves. You go, oh God, I put a lot of this stuff up. You know what I mean? So that was my reason for . . . I only bought things that sold in the grocery store. I made money. I just made money on paper by the fact that somehow I got a statement, I guess. Even though I had the certificate, I still got a statement. I could see that there was more money in the statement. I don't even know if I got it monthly back then. It might have been quarterly. I was getting capital appreciation is what I call it - dividends.

Back in those days you couldn't reinvest your dividends. You had to take them. They sent you a check. Should have saved some. That antique $2 check might be worth 15 cents, might be worth $3 today. Anyway, so I knew I was . . . I knew I was doing okay. I wasn't making no comparison of myself to anybody else. All I knew is, I didn't do anything and I got more money. I wasn't spending it ever, but the value, my worth, was going up.

I did share dealings with my dad some, but he didn't have the interest, you know. I know this now because I'm old, you know. He died when he was 60 so once you get older, you just kind of plowed along and do your stuff, you know. I shared it with mom some because she was around a lot longer, you know. I think we bought a few stocks together. I told her to buy a couple stocks or whatever. You know, we did . . . we sort of jointly bought some.

As a side story, P&C went public during that point in our family's time. It only had about 25 - less than 30 stores for sure. George Smart was the guy's name that took them public and he . . . no, Smart was just a high ranking upstate guy. There was a really bright guy who bought retail. He recognized that my father was a store manager then. He allowed the store managers to participate in the Offering. Now, you know, I'm sure he took care of George Smart, but he did all of them. They got something anyway. Boy, you can't imagine how - it's a long, long story about how they grew unbelievably. They were taken over at least three times. And the last time at some point in time, they squeezed out the top guy from P&C. He made a deal with them. He was a smart guy. He knew up front what the deal was gonna be. He was gonna be eliminated so he made a deal with them. Like he stayed 3 years, 5 years. I don't know. He stayed X number of years and ran the company, you know. And they probably were there to move him one way or the other. I don't know that much about things like that, you know. But anyway, he stayed a few years after it was sold.

So we made a lot of money. My brother could tell you exactly because I got . . . we could buy it, too. Not an offering price, but we could buy it like right away, without too much, I mean, through the company or something. You know what I mean? So I bought some for my brother and gave it to him. He gave me the money and I gave him the stock. He still has, believe it or not, to this day he still has a great portion of it. Because he's, you know, he's made a lot of money on his own. He doesn't have to worry about that stock market. Whether it goes up or down or whatever the hell it does.

But at any rate, where was I? Oh yeah, we put . . . P&C, this is P&C, that's what it began as. And it ended for me as Pneumo Dynamics, I think. They made undercarriages for airplanes. They bought the company for cash flow because you didn't sell a lot of undercarriages, you know what I mean? They wanted to have money coming in on a regular basis so they bought the P&C company for cash flow. And my guess is they probably wrung the shit out of it because they were interested in making undercarriages for airplanes. I don't know.

So as I look back on it, my parents planned well financially for their senior years. I never looked at it quite that way till now. When my father died, there was a mortgage on the house. I think it was . . .

it was certainly less than $150 a month in the 70's. We had just moved next door - a farm house I was raised in. Had a pasture. We took over the pasture and made it a yard and home and all that, you know. My dad even set my grandmom Davis up on our land in a trailer once Marty finished Le Moyne and left my granddad's home to be on his own. She did well there at our place and made it to 94 years old. So my brother and I had this talk. I was working on construction when dad died and the P&C stock was . . . we had had different companies. And he knew about it because I just told you. He had some that I gave . . . I didn't give to him, but he bought it through me. And he said to me . . . or we agreed instantly that there was no need to sell that stock which my mother owned so as to pay off her mortgage so it was just about equal - what was on the mortgage and what the stock value was. After that, it went nuts. It went really crazy after that period of time. So we kissed the ground we walked on that we didn't sell that crap to pay off the mortgage and we both agreed. I told him . . . I had just started construction. I didn't understand about layoffs and not working, but I got to work quite a bit when they were building the nuclear power plant so it wasn't . . . my mother could take care of her expenses anyway. Cover the monthly house payment and the bills. She didn't have to . . . she wasn't concerned about the payment.

Some people wonder about, back then, environmentalists or whoever demonstrating or disrupting our progress on the huge nuclear plant towers – the cones. All I can tell you locally is, if they did it in downtown Scriba, they were not noticeable. Though, I can just tell you this about the town, because my grandfather was a Supervisor of the town in his day, and my father was the Justice of the Peace of the town in his day. The town welcomed the nuclear power plants with open arms. The electric energy outfit wanted to build on the shore because of the water. The Lake could . . . you had to cool that son of a bitch. That's what the water's for. You got to cool that through that cooling tower or the water's got to get cooled. So the town . . . I can remember a guy that made little signs, wooden signs for the front of cars. I can't tell you the year, but "Scriba, the town with a big future" was the plate. I mean, that was a lot of years ago. Obviously, he was quite mistaken.

But any rate, it was . . . when I left Scriba, my whole tax bill - town, county, school - in New York State was not $1,000 a year. And that's, I'll say 15, I'll say closer to 20 years now. But even back then, only had 2 cones while we got 3 now. That electric utility business tax contribution helped us all out, big time. I don't know how wide their service area is; whether it includes Syracuse, which would be a safe bet. The grid is what it is. They talk about the grid. I don't know what it is.

Here's another side story on my dad. He's Justice of the Peace for longer than . . . I still get his pension. This is . . . he was Justice of the Peace for many, many, many years. Because his father-in-law was the Supervisor at one time and his father-in-law was also the meat marker owner - it's a small town. This is not hard to figure out. It was not passed on in the family. You have to get elected. Back in those days when my father was on the Town Board, he was the Justice. Justices were part of the Town Board. They've since done away with that. They don't want the law being conflicting with the, you know. I want to say it this way. This is about me and not about him. It's prestigious. I don't think the money was a great deal of bearing on it, even though the money . . . dad certainly spent it you know. He didn't give it back to the town, but I don't think it was much. He held Court in our house. It was no building to hold Court in. He came in the house, married people in our house. Did that for . . . I told you in the 1960's we moved into a new house. I used to be, I was the best . . . I was not the best man but I guess I was . . . I had to sign the document for some people sometimes since nobody else was handy. Can't think of what you call that.

My point was, when dad got his pension, there was an option on it. You could pass it on to somebody. He would pass it on to my mother.

He said to me, "I'll pass this on to you if you promise to give it to your mother".

Well, you get a lower pay out with that option. I lose a lot because they knew that, what do they call that system the insurance companies got? He lost a lot by it going to me after him because it was a lot smaller. $40 bucks a month I get. Tickles me. I love it. I can't help it.

I had a friend who I told you about. This lady who said my . . . says my mother didn't do me any favors. Her father used to say about me, because he worked for my dad. They worked together; he worked in the Davis Market. Then he left and went with the P&C chain. He was influential in getting my father a job when he closed the Davis Market store so they were really close. He used to say this about . . . he was a meat manager and I would work in the grocery stuff. He worked as meat manager and he used to say this about me: "He hates to lie." And I do hate to lie. I'm better at it now, but when I was younger, I still don't like to lie.

He used to say that about me, "He hates to lie."

Now, here's a piece about me that might gonna be a comedy skit. I told you about hating reading, and my struggle with it. Bad! However, I've always been able to read the newspaper. I don't know if this is true or not but I went through a match situation where I'd have a few women I could scope out about to see how well I'd get along with them. One woman told me a lot of years ago that the newspaper's written to a fourth grade level. So I take that to heart. I don't know if it is or not. I know . . . I know my eyes don't function like a normal person's eyes because of the fact that my eye doctor is able to bill Medicare in such a way that it approves payment for my eye exams once a year. So there's something with my eyes. I just don't know.

For example, I reverse letters. I was talking a while back about the stock symbols, you know. Sometimes I, if it's . . . we'll just make it easy - A, B, C. Sometimes I put down A, C, B. When I punch it in, on the pad, the keypad. I punch it in wrong so I have to go back and find the gd thing again and see what I can do about it. Yup. Lots of things I do even today involve pictures. Like if you look at the New York Times today, and you look at the Broadway shows. In the little box there on the bottom, there's not many pictures, but usually on the page there's pictures of the . . . and sometimes I go the movies today and don't even know what I'm gonna see. I just walk in front of the boards and go "Hey, I think I'll see that", you know. Since I don't care what you call it – dyslexia? - doesn't matter to me. All I know is that maybe it's . . . I'm defeated before I start. All I can tell you is that when it comes to the printed page, with the exception of the newspaper, I give up.

As for research and reports with my stocks, I used none of that so as not to read stuff. I just bought things as I said earlier that I was familiar with. There's not much fine print on a statement really. You know; you get the company's name in there and you got to know the name in order to buy the gd thing. It's generally, I think they are for the most part not perfectly, but they're listed alphabetically so you know the beginning's gonna be the beginning of the alphabet and whatever's on there. Not too hard if you got eight stocks. Not too hard what the first one might be and what the last one. I don't know. I said to you, I just don't . . . all I know is . . . I'll just tell you another story because that's easiest for me to do.

I knew this person who had a fan problem. She needed a fan and she was kind of like desperate. So I went, bought her a fan. I think I might have been at her house so at least I didn't go far from somewhere else. But at any rate I got the fan. Brought it back to her house. Not a big expense, you know. $20, $15, $25, somewhere in there. So she . . . it's in a box and, open the box and it's a pedestal of parts; about no more than 6 pieces fell out. I said, "I'll see you later"! She knows me well enough to know that I wasn't trying not to help her. That I am not gonna pick up those instructions and try to figure out what's going on with them 6 pieces. That's just the way . . . my favorite one of my sayings came from Bill Clinton. It's all about what your definition of "is" is. And if nobody remembers that, I could refresh you, but if you remember, you can fill it in however you wanted to. That's the way life is. It's all about your definition of what "is" is. To me, the printed page is not where I'm gonna go. I've been able to cope with the paper for all my life that I've been here. If it's written to a fourth grade level, I'm able to deal with that. It's if written to a tenth grade level, I'm selling myself short. That's all I can tell you.

I subscribed to the Wall Street Journal. I don't read it hardly at all. As a matter of fact, I stopped subscribing to it because of the fact that I had too much trouble with the whole thing. To be perfectly honest with you, I liked lots of it, but I don't need to get two papers a day. I don't read well so I eliminated the Wall Street Journal easily and stay with my local paper for local stuff.

I need to add something to my not really using tools to pick my stocks, just buying stuff I knew sold good. There's a book that a guy wrote in 1989 . . . saw in the newspaper, the Syracuse newspaper I think because I never had any other paper as an adult. Only time I ever got the New York Times was when I was in high school. Somewhere in a newspaper in upstate New York, there was a little article about this book that was coming out. It was gonna have perks that companies would give you if you owned their stock. So I thought that would be really nice. I like free stuff, no matter what it is hardly. "The 100 best stocks to own in America" by Gene Walden - just like the bookstore, Walden bookstore, I think.

I had a decent portfolio on the little things that I had bought. By then I was 47 and had been dabbling on my own, though I have no accurate memory of the value of my total stocks when I latched on to this book which was going to point me to the free stuff. I've had a few people ask me what I had by then. The only way I can tell you that balance is, as a general rule, I don't think I've put a lot of money into the whole thing. You know, I've put money in each time I bought a new stock, perhaps, but that hasn't happened in years. I haven't put any money in anything. It's just grown.

First, I have to tell you this because I love to tell these little things which might only be memorable for me. But none the less, I want to say it anyway. I was with my mother in the mall in Syracuse - Great Northern Mall it was called back then. I don't know what it's called now, but it was called Great Northern Mall back then. I had mentioned to her that I wanted to go to the bookstore. As a matter of fact, you went to the Walden bookstore to buy a book because that's all there was for buying books. So they had it and probably she went shopping somewhere else. I had just re-joined her and so I told her I bought the book. I probably showed it to her.

And she said, "You must have wanted that really bad."

Because I wouldn't never spend money on any hardcover book. I would even go further to say that's probably the only hardcover book I ever bought. I said, "Yea,I did." I said, "It's going . . . that's got stuff in there about you can own companies and get gifts from them because you own the company". So I told her I just like to see what I can get from a company. That's true. She knew me so well. And she knew my different rough times at every stage of my growing up.

She died of Lymphoma in 1990. She dealt with it a long time, never got any help. My brother and I took care of her at the end of her life when he was living in New York so we were able to get her in NY Sloan Kettering Medical Center. So in New York doctors said we should treat this disease. And in Oswego, the doctors said whether treated or not treated, same result. So she chose not to treat it.

And as time went on, the local doctor said to her, actually said to both of us, "You've really tolerated this lymphoma really well".

And this is like 10 or 12 years after the first development of the cancer. No side effects. She just dealt with it and went home, went on with her life as if nothing was happening. So then the last 10 months of her life were really the hardest for me of my entire life.

You know, my brother's gone off and got the job in New York City, so he's way over there. And I'm living at home and I took care of her. And I really felt responsible for her. So the thing that made the last 10 months of her life so hard for me was it didn't really appear to me to be very hard, but what I've decided about my life now is that I really have a short patience span. I felt like I wasn't doing it justice. I actually went to see a priest. He gave me that bs story about you doing the best you can...

"I'm sure you'll be fine" and all that, but...

As it progressed . . . later I figured this out. I don't like to talk about myself as a worker. I like to think that wherever I worked, I had a fairly decent time. As I look back on it, if I wasn't having a decent time, I didn't think about it at the time, but now that I look back on it, I just left. I didn't leave many times, but when I decided it was time for me to go, I just left. Now that's not to say the money was not always important to me. That's what it boils down to. I made decent money thanks to unionism, no matter what I did. So my point in having fun on the job is that I was not used to having to do anything hard or inconvenient. And that period of taking care of my mom really pushed me to do things way out of my comfort zone. I had lived a charmed life so to speak, up until then, in many ways. 13 years I stayed with her and seeing her go down was just really hard. All of it was hard.

Back to the best book I ever could have bumped into. Marriott stock is the one I remember the most. Marriott gave you half price for corporate owned hotels. So you went to a Marriott hotel that was corporate owned and the price was . . . the cost back then $60 bucks. You got it for $30. I think in some cases there were minimums, but for the most part I don't believe I ever bought enough shares. I probably bought enough shares if it says it in his book to get the stock.

Now my new stock purchases came out of my pocket. I was not a Trader. I didn't . . . I didn't for years and years . . . I never sold nothing. Nothing. Yeah. For years and years I never sold anything. I stayed a steady small size buyer. But I'd been doing that before buying the book. You know, the little things like Fay's Drugs. I just told you about them - turned into Rite Aid. I owned that already, which was in the book. So Jello and those name brands, which turned out to be in the book, I owned all those stocks on my own with no help. Most were on the grocery store shelves as high volume sellers. An exception was Fays drug stores. I'll tell you why. Because it grew and grew. It was a little . . . it was a Syracuse area drugstore and it kept opening up stores all the time. See, I depended on what I was observing. I had a friend who managed one of their stores in Oswego and I asked him. I said, I said,

"You know, it looks like it's growing, a lot of stores opening up".

He was, "Sure is", you know.

I didn't realize this had become sort of an obsession or laser focus in my world, but I had to do something useful. I didn't know anything. I couldn't build a house. So . . . and I can say this today, I can't tell you what my motivation was in my younger years. I'd have to think about that, because I don't really know, but today I call it my hobby to this day. That's what I call it, to this day.

I can tell you this book was an asset because I still own some of these companies today. I can, you know, I'd tell you if you want to. I glance here in the book at one just got taken over and one that I still own that actually Cook took over . . . I see two that I just owned until one of them got taken over, just checking off the list charts here, and I still own AnheuserBusch today. You know, so but a lot of them like, I own VF, Vanity Fair. That's . . . they make clothes and they're based up in North Carolina. I had that a long time and I own, I told you Sherwin Williams I still own to this day. Remember, we did not sell paint in the grocery store. So I'd have never found that without this book. Another one I own here on this author's list, C R Beard, Bard, whatever it's called.

When I moved down here twenty years ago, people who wanted to become your financial advisor used to put on little groups. They called them seminars, early on they called them that. I used to go to those often when I came down here. Mostly because I wanted somebody to analyze my portfolio, for free of course, and a lot of people did that back then. They analyze your portfolio and one of the first ones who ever analyzed was, I don't know who it was, but he said all you own is retail stuff. So I had to make some adjustment. But I didn't hire him. I just decided, well, I got to look at this differently. I got time to do that instead of paying him to do it.

I can tell you this also. My mother was born in 1917 and she died at 73. And she died in . . . yeah, I think she might have been sick maybe at the time I bought the book, 1989. She died in a hospital but she was only there a couple days. I . . . when she was first diagnosed with this situation, I mean, not when she was diagnosed, but when things took a turn for the worst, right? I was out of work so it wasn't any problem. I just stayed home and took care of her. As it began, it . . . I didn't get a lot of work out of the Union Hall when they weren't doing time/materials/cost plus work because I'm not a rough and tumble kind of worker, and all that kind of stuff. I look at it that way now. I have to make a joke about it. I'm not very personable. They usually kept me in unemployment. You know, they usually, I mean, I was in my late 40's; I didn't really have any expenses so the smaller income did not set me back. My mom paid the mortgage; I never paid rent. My nights of getting drunk here and there were behind me. Even the Speedway, once my dad died, it had tapered off by the time I was in my . . . maybe, I think, before my dad died, I had stopped but anyway just, it's a good way to say it. Around the time my dad died, I'd stopped going. I just, because I hope you like the humorous part. This is just the truth of the way I thought about it. I was going up the Speedway; taking my cooler with the vodka and orange juice in it; getting really drunk. So I decided I would just eliminate going into the racetrack. Just go to a bar and do that. Same end result. You know, I can't tell you why I think that way, but that's just a factual thing – my world.

After my mom died, my routines were really new for me. My mom left the house to me, not me and my brother. And he was OK with that. He was doing real well on his own. Finally when I wanted to spend an overnight with a girlfriend, she could come over to my house for a change. I mean, I very rarely went to anybody else's house when my parents were alive anyway. I'm sure I did. Stayed and get up in the morning and get out. But I . . . I'm not a social critter. I mean, I needed private time with someone but I did not need the overnight stuff. I've come to . . . I've come to think about myself. An afternoon and early night date at her place was all I needed. What can I say? It's just me.

As far as retirement, again, someone looking out for me. It was easy. It was an easy choice that they . . . that they want to make . . . the

Union wants to make it easy for you at that point in life because at 55 years old as a laborer, you're not as productive as they want you to be. A lot of people stay around longer. Don't get me wrong, but in my case, I wasn't getting enough work to talk about - just staying above water with the work to get unemployment. It was an obvious thing for me to just, to just end it.

As far as long term planning before or even then about retiring at an early age, to be perfectly honest with you, I didn't plan a thing. I was flying blind. And I just took one event as it came after another. As I think about it right now, just a little thing I know about myself, for whatever reason, is that I don't like inconvenience. The work was, the work was too hard to get for me. It was an inconvenience. I had to beg and plead with the Union. I don't do that very well either obviously so I just . . . it was time for me to end it.

I've only had two jobs as I've told you. I tell this story often about myself. There may be parts of this I've already said to you. I had a psychologist that I really liked.

He put me on disability because he told me, "You need time off". You shouldn't be working. You got to be on disability".

So I thought that was a fine thing because I could get disability, you know. So I had this opportunity when I was on disability to go on construction, whatever the time frame is. They're building this nuclear power plant I told you about coming to town. You worked all the time, almost like a factory job you know. You never went home. So I told him - I went back to see him and told him about my opportunity to go on construction though I hated to give up the P&C grocery thing for, you know, because they've . . . I've been there a long time and he said you're not disabled from construction; you're disabled from the P&C job. You can go on construction and still get your disability. I did that so he must have wrote it up that way. I don't think I would engineer it, you know, so I did that.

Came time when the disability was up, I guess. I had to make a choice. My father was still alive. I can tell you that - 1977. He knew

I was working on construction. He knew my circumstance. He died same year. But whenever this time frame was, he was still alive. And he said to me - he became a supervisor; like he had twelve stores he had to go visit, oversee - regional supervisor. That's what he was. So he was on disability too at that time. As a matter of fact, you know, because he wasn't getting along very well, because he didn't die very much after that, he died pretty soon.

And he said to me about the grocery business. "It doesn't get any better." That's what he said. He reminded me about "Harold Brown will take good care of you".

So I made a decision to quit. My way I quit was, I went to the grocery store while I was also working construction. I told them I had two weeks vacation coming and to consider that my two weeks notice. I was finished. So we didn't leave on very good terms. But back to the way I seem to see things. It was more convenient one way than it was the other way. My father instilled into me, it wasn't gonna get any better. Harold Brown by the way is a friend of mine and he was a . . . he used to work part time for my dad before he went on construction. He was in with the Union goings on.

For a lot of years after my mother passed away in 1990 I had, I guess what people called it, or I called it or whatever you want to call it, I had an ongoing garage sale. This would have been like taking me through from 50 – 55 when I was not getting a lot of Union work and I had time on my hands. No master plan. I was fortunate enough or unfortunate enough to live on a main artery. Route 104 is like a main highway east and west. Goes across the state of New York up on the top. Probably traffic is all alleviated now some because of the Throughway. The Throughway is still there but 104 still got a lot of traffic. So I decided I'd have a garage sale. We had a two car garage and a patio over - covered patio over one end of it - ranch house, you know. It was concrete there up to the garages. Remember, I had a full, crammed packed basement inventory in rows and aisles from my mom, the hoarder.

So I put some stuff out. I never forget, the first year the garage was kind of full. I don't know why that was but it was. So I pushed all the stuff back towards the wall and kind of made a little line in the sand and put some things out for sale. And then I remember that I came to realize . . . I came to realize that I wasn't ready to part with anything. I priced everything really high. I wasn't doing that consciously. They have a thing now if you ever watch the television. There's a guy, couple of guys that go around the country. Their sellers are frequently attached to their goods, you know. Well, I was attached to it all. I put it out there even though I didn't think I was attached. So I didn't sell much the first year. I probably didn't sell much for the first 2 or 3 years. I just had retail in my blood and also loved that cash, no matter how small, trickling in. I don't know. But as time went on, I got better at it. I reduced things every week so I could get rid of it, you know. All the things I saw my dad do for so many years. But my goal was to get rid of it so I did that. And I got rid of quite a bit.

So I decided, I have a NY acquaintance who I still have today. She is a Southern born lady. She retired early and went to Alabama to be closer to her sister. Then she decided to work a bit longer. She took a job as a, like a supervisor for classrooms of pre-school – pre-thing the government supports. So I thought, well it's time to put my house on the market so I can get out of this snow. So . . . it took me about certainly over a year to sell it. Because there again, hey, I wanted a dollar number and I wanted that number. My realtor gave me a number. I didn't get it from him. However I was not depending on this sale price to be the windfall which would fund my retirement. I think I'd had enough faith in this hobby of mine by then that I was doing all right with this. I don't even recall the sale price. I can't even - I can't even tell you what I did with the sale money. Again, I had no plan. I am very simple. One step at a time.

I know some of it I put in the market. You know, the cash I got out of the house. I know I did that. Maybe I put it all in the market. So maybe I could say that. Yeah, maybe I did. I can't even tell you what I did with it. I know I didn't . . . I always considered myself poor. More because I think people are rich who can sell their skills some to somebody so they hire them. I was really tough to get hired. I needed convenience. I've grown to understand that.

In fact I do not even have a history track of how much my stock accounts increased every 5 years or 10 years so I have no bench marks. I always just had a number that I wanted to have. I wanted to have a million dollars. I wanted to see that number be a million dollars on the . . . on the, not even then, no computer existed. I wanted that statement to come. There was a program called something about a millionaire years ago. Maybe I got it from there. I don't know where I got it from but I had that number in my head. A million was just a fun fantasy for me. I was not planning anything. It is a hobby so I picked something out of the air. I remember the guy's name on the TV show, John Beresford Tipton. I got it from them, whenever that was on. I have no idea really. I don't know why I picked it up. Michael Anthony delivered the check. Tipton's name came right to mind because he's the guy I wanted to match. The delivery guy's name was harder to recall.

Oddly enough, I never had the slightest belief that I would even really grow a pile of money. I never did. I didn't never think it would come anywhere near a million. I had a . . . I don't know. I'm just gonna call it an epiphany. I don't know what that means really but I came to realize that, some point in time, that I just structure things. Like how I have made money or what times I've made money. I've been raised a Republican all my life. I'm still a registered Republican; however, the most money I - it goes back a while. That's why I'm trying to tell you like it is. I came to realize when Bill Clinton was in power for his 8 years, in which I never voted for him, I made more money than I had ever made in the stock market. I can't tell you a number but I could realize that I had made a lot of money during those 8 years when he was the President of the United States. So when he went out of office, whether I consciously thought I was comfortable or not, I don't know but I didn't have a million dollars. I just know I did . . . I did really well.

I can't tell you what the number was but I was happy that I had done really well. This was the 90's.

So then Mr. Bush comes into power, handed a beautiful plate of food. No debt! The Country didn't even have any gd debt, you know. So I thought, hey I voted for him the first time because he was a Republican. I was still in Scriba when he got in the first time. I voted at the little town. So sometime after he was in, I left.

I came to stay with my lady friend in Alabama but I couldn't stand it. Just I was discomforted again. Maybe make that the title of my story here. I left Alabama and came over here to the Atlantic Ocean beach since my brother has a place I could live and not cost me. I had no roots, and I had no practice ever living in my own place, alone, away from home. I would have liked for that Alabama trial attempt to settle, to have worked out better, I thought. I didn't do a lot to help it. And I kept telling her that I wanted us to live together. So she didn't work at it fast enough, you know. She's still that way today. She's just . . . she putters more about things than she does get them done.

So that's all right but I wasn't patient enough. So I left over there. I can even tell you when it was. It was Master's golf weekend in Augusta because I had to go from Alabama to the beach through Augusta, GA. So in my little pea brain that I live in, my world, I thought this will be really good. I'll stop in Augusta. I'll walk around that golf course I've seen on the television for a lot of years, you know. It will be nice. I don't want to see a Player. I wasn't there to see any game. I just want to see those flowers and all that stuff I had seen on the television. So I got to Augusta. I'm gonna say at 3 or 4 o'clock in the afternoon - late in the day. The parking lot was pretty well empty. You know, people had gone whatever for whatever reason. Big name guys had gone off or whatever so I thought this is gonna be great. Get out of my car. A guy rolled up in a golf cart and told me I owed him $5 to park. I said you got to be kidding me. I said look at this place. There's nobody here. And he says he's a good employee. If it were me, I'd have just drove my cart away and said, "You're right. Park over here". But he insisted on $5. I didn't want to give it to him so I drove around for a little while. I did find a place to park for free, thank god. I don't know how much money I had in my checking account then, or how much cash I had on me; and I didn't owe anybody any money, not a soul. Nonetheless, he was not going to get my $5. I don't owe anybody any money today except what's on the credit card. I had enough that I wasn't worried though it was not a million dollar portfolio for sure. The parking lot was empty. I mean really empty. It was obvious. I didn't have to be a rocket scientist that it wasn't gonna fill up after I got in there. You know? It wasn't . . . it was just the principle of the thing. So I found a parking place. To make matters worse to even tell you, I parked for free; I went to the gate.

I was driving my slick Bonneville, Pontiac Bonneville. Paid cash for it. Can't recall the price. Whatever the number was with a tradein. It didn't matter to me. I saved $3000 a year every year. I put it in a special account so I could buy a car. I pay myself first, this special savings account, instead of paying the bank with interest afterwards. A long time ago I sent away for a . . . it was in the . . . what is it? "Popular Science" or something like, something science. Anyway, it was in the little ads in the back.

"How to save 25% buying a new car."

Yeah. And I sent them something, $2, $5. I wrote out the form and sent them the money they wanted. I wanted to know how to buy a car.

They sent me a note which came back, "Pay cash".

So that seemed logical to me. That's what I started to do. I can't remember being agitated with my having to buy such a simple solution but I am sure I was quite put out.

So I go to the Augusta gate thinking I can just pay and go in. Yes! I was willing to pay to go in. They won't take my money. The tickets for the round that day are sold out. So no matter what you do, you can't get in. Even if you try to convince them that you want to get in. They're good employees, too. So I didn't get in. I came over here and I haven't been back to Augusta since but I should be. I should buy a ticket and go in.

Anyway, why did that come up? Oh, because I left Alabama and I came over here to the Atlantic coast. That's the year I came over here. I moved into my brother's place, like a drifter or carpetbagger. I mean I had no idea I would be there as long as I was. Leaving home really threw me off. The situation with his condo was, when I got there, his children were either employed working really hard or else they had kids. They might come down for one week in the summer. It was three of them. They might come down and use it for one week in the summer. So I had those 2 units right here across the street from his condo location. These 2 units in here that I owned still in this building, I was using for rental property. I owned those units long before I left Oswego. That's what I did with my rental property when I had my IRS rental property exchange deal that I told you about. I rolled it over. I rolled it over and bought a unit in here to rent.

When one of Marty's grandkids would come down, I would have to evacuate. You might think I would move into my rental condo by taking it off the rental program for a few weeks. Absolutely not. I bought them to make money, not for me to live in, when I had my brother's place for almost free. I would pack up my junk; sometimes maybe go to Alabama. Sometimes I'd rent a motel room for a week; stay there, you know. Simple. Convenient. Cheap. My world. Then when they left, I'd cart my shit over and put it back there. It's eye opening to hear myself say this but I transferred back and forth for a number of years, a number of years – like about 10 to 13 years I guess maybe. Whatever I had to do, I just did it. Plodding along. Never had my own place.

About 7 years ago is the first time I ever had a real place of my own from when I left home – 1998 to 2012. I can remember taking my stuff out of my fill-in condo here and getting a cart from downstairs and walking over there with that cart - carrying it myself upstairs. You talk about what I had? Possessions? I told you I was just about living out of my trunk. I can tell you what I had, not specifically. You don't need to hear that. Let me put it this way. I never had a third cart. Two carts would take it. Actually if you want to know the truth, moving back and forth was great for me because if you move something one year, then move it the next year, it was time for me to throw that away. So I just got rid of it. I didn't use it for the whole year so no sense in toting it back and forth. So I threw a lot of stuff away; didn't amount to nothing.

I got more crap now then I've ever had, here in this one bedroom condo I've owned for 6 or 7 years. This is like I've really made it. I'm living a life of luxury for a poor student from Scriba. I been . . . I'm sure this is true because I've heard it about myself. I don't agree with it but I probably am . . . commitment's a hard word for me. I don't do it well. I try to avoid commitment. So if I don't own anything, I don't commit to anything. I had a person kept telling me, I should have something.

"It would be a good idea to own something. You should have your own place."

So . . . you know I have to say. Everything I learn in life, I learn from what I hear. It also takes a long time for me to understand that what somebody's telling me is probably the truth and I need to hear it and I should act. I should act on it so it took me a long time to act on the notion that I should have something. I didn't see any need to have anything.

As I've aged now, I can tell you that I could never do what I did before - cart my stuff with a cart from over there; take it up stairs; bring it downstairs. To me then it was just nothing. Just what I did. Like having breakfast or whatever you do. It's just what I did. I didn't realize it was a way for me to stay connected to my brother. I wrote him a check for being over there. I mean, we are close but we are not close. We discussed Mullanisms, so whatever it is. He's what he is and I'm what I am. We are what we are and we get along well. That's a good thing I think.

I guess my rental venture went like this. I rolled over my Oswego units to a two bedroom unit here. I did so well the first year with the two bedroom part of it, I took over the adjoining efficiency. It so happened, the guy who sold me the two bedroom was a psychologist by trade. I never met him. He owned the efficiency that was attached to my two bedroom. So I kept in touch with him until I convinced him to sell that to me because I thought it would be a better rental if I had 2 connecting units. Well, that didn't work, but I did own it, you know.

I only had a small mortgage on it because I - well, what I did was. Here's how it went with the banker. Just so I can tell you that real story. Actually, I had a big mortgage on the extra unit I bought from him. I only had a small mortgage on the two bedroom. I didn't have much of a mortgage. And I negotiated with the same banker when I bought the efficiency. I explained to the banker that whatever he did for me and however I got the loan, whatever was happening, that he . . . he didn't have much invested in it, you know. In my two bedroom he didn't have much invested in it so what I wanted to do was buy the efficiency with no money and transfer the debt from the little loan I had to the combined units. Then I would have one larger mortgage for the whole thing. That took a little bit of convincing to get him to do that but he was kind enough or I was persuasive enough or whatever so I wound up with a small unit that they held the mortgage on with a big payment on the smaller unit and I owned the other one out right.

Now I have to keep reiterating, I never felt myself wealthy until I had a number, until I got a statement with my fantasy number on it. All the other things were just things I did because I could do them or I was able to do and I obviously didn't do rentals very well because today I have none. I never considered real estate to be a part of my portfolio. It was the John Beresford Tipton number from my fantasy which playfully might enable me to consider myself wealthy.

My portfolio is what they call my stock. As life goes, I obviously didn't do rentals very well. It would be crazy for me to ever think about trying that again. Overall I lost miserably because my definition of loss and other people's is different. First off, I didn't make any money so that to me is a loss. So even if it was flat, I lost because I didn't . . . nothing appreciated. I didn't make anything on the investment for the rental. Then I didn't make anything when I sold it. There's other ways for me to lose money, too; not just real estate!

Bear markets - I can't say consciously that I ever had a real bad time with anything until George W. left office. It was election in 2008 so it was '09 when it . . . it was at its worst at the end of '08. A great thing to mention is that I was not hurt by the tech bust. To this day, don't know anything about tech. And back then I didn't know anything about tech except. The way I do these things is, you have to keep increasing your dividend every year for a minimum of 7 to 10 years. Tech wasn't paying any dividends back then so I didn't own any of those. I got hurt in the 90's but not majorly.

I can tell you in '08; I'd have been 66. I'd already survived the tech bust - without any pain to speak of, believe me. I never sold a thing or did nothing. I didn't even . . . I hate to say it. I didn't even blink. So in 2008 in the late summer and early fall, I was about, I'm gonna say $3,000 to $6,000 from having the statement come that would be a $1,000,000 which I was really looking forward to. That's the . . . and when you get there, it takes a lot of years. It's unbelievable. It's coming. It's like, I can't describe it. So then George W. decided that Bill Clinton changed some laws in his time to make mortgages get easier so it was his fault that the housing market went to hell. Since after 8 years, George W. mentioned the fact that the god damn thing wasn't right for 8 years, you know. So I lost a lot. If you want to know numbers, I'll tell you. $300,000 just prior to getting my statement of a lifetime with my number on it. It . . . it really upset me. I can . . . I know that. I don't know how much it upset me but it was bothering me a lot. And it was like . . . I never shared a number with anybody back then – never. Nobody knew anything about my assets.

I've saved that oh so close statement ever since with the number on it showing that I had almost reached my fantasy number. I don't know where it is now. You have to . . . you know, when I'm talking like this about myself, I have to realize that's the reason I had to grow up - the reason I did grow up. Because between moving down here, and living through the thing, I know I can't change the world. I'm never gonna and it's my policy. I try not to . . . I try not to be concerned on anything that doesn't affect my life. So because the way I run my life, probably more often than not, there's not very many things that affect my life very much. The way I run my life is, I want to use the word singularly. I try to . . . people that are . . . have been really good to me and have stuck with me for whatever reason, I try to never forget those people and thank them every time I . . . that's another good reason for me telling this story about myself.

It's only been in the last few years, I get to put a name on it. I've had to learn the word thank you. Because I just expected I was going to get it from childhood. The town that I grew up in was easy for me. Just happened. I never . . . whether I could read or write didn't make any difference, you know. I could have a job and I could work and do those things. But I try to go out of my way to say thank you to lots of people now and I probably don't do it nearly as well as anybody else does but I do it better than I've ever done.

So I guess you could say that being mindful of being grateful makes living my life easier. I just know that. You know, the more people you . . . I call it petting the dog the wrong way. The more people you alienate, you pet the dog the wrong way. You never want to pet the dog the wrong way. The dog only likes front to back, not against the coat layer. Only good to pet one way so that's just what's happened - for reasons that are beyond my realm of comprehension. It's just my life that I have lived. Nothing I sat down and said now I can do this and this and this. I think people who are educated probably do that in some sense, when they got a diploma to sell. They got some sense that makes value for them, for them to be. I don't have that.

My friend who I just talked about from the South, I'm sure I was crying to her about my huge, huge loss. She's got to have shoulders like, that are like astronautical.

She said to me, "Are the stocks doing what you bought them for?"

Because I had preached to her about buying stocks to pay dividends and raise their dividends. I said, "Yea, most of them. A few aren't", and I've pared those that aren't doing now what I wanted them to do. I've taken, I think, I probably took profits the fact that I had them for so long. I basically had gotten rid of most of them because 2 things happened. Either a company eliminated their – 3 things happened. Either a company cut their dividend or a company eliminated their dividend for a short period of time – 3 or 4 years.

And banks . . . what banks did, which is a wonderful business story to me or what a lot of companies did, because I really like this. This is a great business story. They paid a penny 4 times a year or a dime or something so they can write in their little annual booklet that they never stopped paying the dividend. They never . . . they've paid a dividend since so long ago. They know that in their mind when they do that. Dividends cost companies money. That's what you have to remember about a little thing I know about the market. Dividends are an expense, a big one. They got a lot of shares out there so I've never said it this way. Never even thought about it but count yourself lucky when you get that dividend because you're riding on somebody's coat tails who's making some money while giving you a little chunk of it. Don't ever give it back to them. Take it.

Contrary to what the professionals say, you know, everybody's, you know, "You have to reinvest your dividend today."

My style is, reinvest your dividend in another company. Let that company treat you nice so you can invest in another company.

So she helped me realize I had done what I wanted to do. You know, if I haven't reached my number, I got to continue to do it my way to the point, you know, as long as a lot of - . There again that's something that those, my word, dirty bastards do - they raise their dividend by a penny so they can write in their little program that we've never stopped paying a dividend. They know things are gonna be good. They're a big company. They know. What's the worst that can happen to them? Is that penny causing them to go out of business? Heck no. They don't have to write zero dividend in the book. They've raised them a penny so a lot of companies I own still raise their dividend a penny. So I still got those companies. So she reminded me I could just stay the course.

I sold off some, I just told you. I never pared really until then. I pared a lot then, you know. They had to go. I can't remember the number but I - if they stopped the dividend, they were out of my world. I didn't want to own them anymore. It ended. I told you. The 2 action extremes was, they paid a penny or they raised a penny. If they didn't . . . uhuh. So when you sell a bunch, you have to do something with the cash so as to put it in some other more profitable companies. And I had never pared like this before. For a lot of years, even before the 2008 crash, a lot of years I had bought another book. I think I've had it that long so then probably I relied on that as my tool. For a long time I kept an eye on this book that had every company in the S&P 500 listed in two pages. It gave me all the information that I wanted to have. I got out of this what I needed to know to buy and rearrange what I owned. I did not do a bunch of research I would have had to read. I just used these columns of figures the two page listing provided - only the numbers part of it. You know, the company name and the numbers part of it – can't recall the book name.

So oddly enough, I finished selling off. I want always . . . for me it's a tax deal. I hate to pay tax on my stocks. I finished selling off in December of '08 when it went down. And it was still going down. In '09 it went down and I think the lowest day was in March of '09. There was a guy on a cable channel who called the day. Who called the day!

"This is the low", he said.

He's passed away now. They mention him often. At any rate I . . . in the beginning of 2009 when I had a lot of money, meaning cash in my stock account, I just started doing what I always did. Buying things in '09; putting cash back in. Consequence was, I accidently bought at the low. Accident, believe me. Not a plan. Just, that's what I've always done. I always was in the market totally, all the time. Never out. So I figured, hey, when I got this money, I'm gonna start putting it in during January. It's first of the year and I don't think I ever . . . I think I had it all in before that date in March that it hit the low. But I . . . I obviously didn't lose a lot at that point in time between January and

March because I'd have a hard time tolerating a further loss deal, you know what I mean? So all those things I bought in early '09, I probably still own. I don't think I ever sold anything. Like I said, I don't do a lot of turnover. I stay for the long haul.

I have to preface this because I want it to be an honest number with you, I inherited some. I inherited from Rusty, a cousin of mine - $174,000. And it was strictly out of the blue because we weren't close. He had the same hobby as me. We'd talk on the phone. He lived in New Hampshire and I lived in Scriba. I used to invite him to come down when he was alive. I said to come down to the beach. "Bring your Aunt Mathilda with you", you know. "Stay a couple weeks. I can book something nice here for you so you can stay." He never did, but anyway, he left me 174 grand; 5% of whatever he owned - whatever 5%, whatever $174,000 was. I was the lowest one on the totem pole and I always . . .

Oh, God. I got to tell the truth. It takes a long time. My father really took to heart his family, even though there was the parents who were dead for a long time. His brothers and sisters were important to him. He was younger. He was one of the younger ones. And as time went on, they died because he was a lot younger than them. So some were in Syracuse who died. So every Memorial Day we went to the Scriba cemetery where my mother's parents' parents (Leger) - because my mother's parents were still alive when I was a kid - where my mother's grandparents were buried. We'd put flowers on their grave and it wasn't a sad moment for my father because he didn't even know them for one thing, those particular in-laws. But then we would drive to Syracuse and put flowers on the graves of his sisters and brothers who had passed away more recently. And it was never sad. It was always . . . yeah, it was a great thing. So I don't know where that piece came in, where ever we are. I just have to say that about, you know, Memorial Day, to me. It's not . . . even though it's harder because my parents are there. Yet I remember that and my father, which was . . . and he had . . . he wanted urns for them. He didn't want to put them in the ground.

We had to buy urns to put them in.

Oh, I know, the added cash inheritance thing got me there. So by March of 2009, part of me felt like I was starting all over; and part of me was encouraged that I still had $700,000 at the market low. I got this $174,000 from Rusty but I still wasn't rich though a $174,000 is a lot of money to me and I didn't earn it. It just like fell from the sky. So I spent $30,000. That's why I went into that urn story with you. I figured since my father . . . we went to those cemeteries in Syracuse. There were a lot of these mausoleums which were in those big Catholic cemeteries where his relatives were buried. I was taken by that, you know, for whatever reason - very impressive. I don't have any idea.

So with that $174,000 gift bundle, I spent some, a lot of money on a mausoleum I directed be erected in the cemetery in Scriba today. And that's where my body's gonna go into when I die. It's just a one grave thing. It's only for me. Stands above the ground. We didn't go elaborate or anything like that. It's just a, it's a marble box that you . . . I learned that doesn't make any difference whether you go into the ground or not since they have to put air vents in those mausoleums. Otherwise they would blow up because of the gas in human bodies. I should have just stuck with the ground. In my case and in Syracuse, when I went around with my father, the graves were just free standing structures on a plot they had, usually for a husband and wife - maybe for kids. That's what they were – a fancy place for a box. Then it's wrote on there that I'm the son of the people who are buried next to me. I only did that because I have a cousin who is into that stuff about genealogy. She told me it's a lot easier if that's on there. But I like to have it on there - I'm the son of etc. That's why I put it on there. On the back of it, it reads, "Thank you, Rusty Dougherty". He's the guy who gave me the money.

So that chunk of money went for my burial stone stuff. I don't remember what else I did. But that was the major expense that I incurred. Then I put what was left of that money into this Schwab portfolio where I had a balanced fund - separate portfolio so I could keep track. When you talk about downturns, we're having one as we speak here, April, 2018 – adjustment. Prior to this downturn, the $174,000, which I spent $30K of, was almost back to a hundred percent. Now it's recovered 80 some percent. But no other help. Just me and my Gene Walden book.

I can still use it now. A lot of the stocks he named are still in existence. Marriott's certainly still in existence. His recommendations are still part of my portfolio - a lot of them. I bought them then and I still own them. I won't say a lot of them. There's a hundred in his book here so I'll go backward. I shouldn't say this because it kind of screws it up. I own Pepsi Cola today. That's in there. I own Genuine Auto Parts today. That's in there. I own Automated Data Processing. That's in there. So I can go through say, 10. That's 3. There's probably 20 – 30 that I still own of his 100.

So big picture, I got out of high school at 20 in 1962. Stayed employed like I told you from 20 till I was 55. Kept plugging away at my hobby. Came down here for the past 20 years to the beach. So let's look at what I am worth today all together. I wanted to mention that $30,000 what I spent. I've given money to a regional community foundation near Scriba. I wanted to count this in my total because they give me interest of whatever I've given them. So I've given them pretty close to $300,000. My portfolio is worth now, the Fidelity portfolio which includes my IRA - that's relatively small but it's . . . I'll say it's a million four. Add stuff that I got; add my mother's inheritance; and it's over, way over, it's closer, it's over 2 million. It's up 80% from . . . I can turn on the computer and tell you an exact number but I just can't come up with that right now. So I don't know what that adds up to but I add that in and certainly well over two million. Yeah, over two million! My number was always a million. However I didn't reach the two million number by mistake. I say I have a hobby. I didn't say by mistake.

My point of all this, you know, is that I'm a little weird. My world. I never had any children and never had a wife but there's no reason that people can't be selfsustaining if they got a document to sell themselves with. Anybody who digs themselves such a big hole that they're in debt, it's because they're not very conscientious of what the hell they're doing. What the hell they're doing! That's all. If you want to end up like that, you can do it or do whatever you want to do. I could talk to you forever. Forget it.

What I would like people, students and adults, to take away from my journey are a couple things. First, the fact that I learned late in life to say thank you. Then again by now, you all know I am a slow learner. But, well I'll tell you, it's really easy for me to say what I think everybody should get from this. However this is not why I'm really doing this. Take me. School failure three times; graduated when I was 20 from high school, and not a discipline issue, mind you. People think that the stock market's a mystery. It isn't a mystery. I'm no detective. I am not bright. If a little brain like mine can figure out the stock market, and do well, and not have any help; if you make a little effort; if you pay as much attention to watching a football game and who's ranked, or what the standings are and all that stuff, you can certainly adjust your focus to end up comfortable, if you give up a football game or two. Now, do I know anything about sports? I don't know where the net goes on the football field. I know nothing about sports and it doesn't affect my life, my comfort, my security, my fear of the future. Never has. Never missed it. I love my hobby. That's a big challenge for me. Things that don't affect my life, I don't pay any attention to. Somebody told me once I live on my own critical path, whatever that is. I know I have to be simple because that is my world. Sports does not . . . like if you ask me who won the Super Bowl last winter as I sit here in April of 2018, all I can tell you is, not New England. Can I tell you who they played? Can't come up with it. I should know it. If I dug around long enough, I probably could. I don't track standings in any sport. Heck, I can not even gain paid entry to the Augusta Master Golf gardens.

I have a friend who has a diploma - lady from Syracuse University. She loves Syracuse University. I lived up there for a long time. There's no professional team except a AA or AAA baseball team. I never could stand to go. On the other hand there's Syracuse University. Has football and basketball. They do pretty well in football again. Since she's dedicated, I pay a little bit of attention to Syracuse University. But other than that . . . I am old so I have seen Dolph Shayes play pro basketball. Two handed set shot artist. Now days, lots of basketball fans know nothing of Dolph or even know what a set shot is. He played for the Syracuse Nationals. And they got bought out and moved by? Look it up on all that fancy computer stuff everyone has!! I know because I lived there, otherwise I'd be in the dark maybe.

I'll tell you something else about sports that you might want to learn today that I know. This could go on a long time, you know. Told you I love to talk. The 24 second clock was invented by the guy who owned the Syracuse Nats, Danny Biasone. He owned it a long time. You wouldn't believe the amount of money he got for that team when it went. I used to know that number but it was preposterous, even by today's standards. It was absolutely nothing. They played in an Arena that only seated, I would guess, 8, 10 would be a stretch, 10,000. I don't think it seated 10,000. It was a really small arena. It was called War Memorial in Syracuse.

Another thing, a lot of people think Jim Boeheim got the Dome built, the Carrier Dome. Jim Boeheim did not get that built. The people that wanted to . . . I can't tell you the people but the reason it got built was because a couple things. They wanted a way to encourage football players to come to Syracuse and play. So they built a dome to protect them from the lousy winter weather – snow all the time. Cost money, too, to clear snow from seats and aisles in an open stadium where they played, Archbold Field. Only one of three stadiums in the world in 1907, built of concrete. I listened a little to stories on that concrete job for the nuclear power plant towers! It seated 40,000 but by the '70's, old age broke down some areas and maybe 25,000 is all they could seat legally by the fire marshall. And the league, the NCAA, was going to demote them from first class to second class – whatever they call that. So they built the Carrier Dome by demolishing Archbold. I mean they really went to town with this. This Dome is the largest domed stadium on any college campus in the Country! I've been in it for a basketball game. They just curtain off the football field and put up the court.

Last Syracuse story. Come on. It's my home town almost. Jim Boeheim was a walk-on for Syracuse University for the varsity basketball team. He comes from a town called Marcellus, not very far from Syracuse. He got a scholarship for his grades so he became a scholarship student and I guess that entails housing. So he was housed with the basketball team. And the rest is history. He turned out to be the second best player on the team. Dave Bing was the best player on the team, from Detroit. They're still close. Now when everybody would go home for Thanksgiving, Boeheim would invite anybody who didn't have the money to go home who was a basketball player or something, to his house for Thanksgiving dinner. He was going home because he lived so close. Now apparently he had a car so he would take them there. I don't think they arrived on their own. The story I heard was, he'd bring them to this house. He wouldn't tell them that his house, his father was an Undertaker where he did business. He lived over the Undertaker operations so Jim Boeheim does have a sense of humor. Anyway, I lived there a long time. That's the only reason I know those things. They were in the newspaper - the Post Standard, whatever level that's written to. And that was the sum total of my reading adventures – the local paper. Still is, here with my local beach Blade. Part of my ritual. So Jim put or helped to put Syracuse on the map. Though I don't think my story will put Scriba on the map. I doubt it. It will be a stretch.

Let me say something really serious about my family story. It's easy to say after all these years. It was easy to say then because it floats right to the top. I was 35. I was with my dad the morning he died. He wasn't himself for months, weeks, I don't know - quite some time. I can't say if it was the disability the Doc put him on. Just that, I can't, you know . . . we been through this thing here. You know probably that's a piece of me that . . . it's the same thing. My father's . . . I think his dependency was a lot on . . . he was a politician in a small town - well recognized. He did really well in the company he worked for. He got to be up there.

After that was gone, it was . . . you know, he went on disability; like maybe a somebody who thought he became a nobody when his public status and roles changed.

As a matter of fact, just as an aside to all this because I don't mind talking about anything much, you know. Like I went with him to the psychologist. I got him to go to the psychologist that I was going to who I just talked about. I think I might have been over that but he was still alive then. Whatever time frame that was. My father went to see him. He told him, you know, he was depressed. At any rate now, I might not have all this just right. I went to see him . . . I went with him to some doctor. Oh no. It wasn't a psychologist. I think I just went to see . . . oh, some doctor. I hate to do this but I don't remember. Anyway the doctor he went to, the doctor about his back, and I went with him. Wasn't anybody I associated with.

The doctor said, "Your pains are not that bad".

You know, he didn't say exactly your pain is not that bad.

He said, "You know, the Xrays and things show me that, you know, you don't have a lot of pain".

Driving the car - he had to drive a lot because he was this district director, you know, but his Doctor said,

"It doesn't look that bad to me". "You know", he said, "You can choose what you want to do. I can do this or that or - "

You can say about some Doctors, if you pay them, they'll do whatever you want them to do. So my father decided, I guess, right there in the office, he wanted to take disability. And I guess I drove him up and back because he was having trouble with his back, too. It was in Syracuse. So on the way home, I just said to him, "You know, maybe it wasn't written in stone yet", but I said, "Are you sure you want to do this, you know; like work, you know, work's been a big thing"? I am not eloquent, and I am still not now.

At any rate, he said, "Yes."

And I'm just gonna make this up. I'm gonna say that was in the Fall. Christmas time, he was dead. Period. So I got a feeling that it was easily predicted. However, when you're living it, it doesn't . . . it doesn't ring your bell until it happens, and you look back.

Why did he die? It's my opinion. They have a saying about opinions. Everybody knows what they are. It's just my opinion. Just pops into my head now, there again, about this. When my father was on the road as a supervisor, he would go to stores where they had merchandise they were marking down. Probably prayed they'd get rid of it. He used to buy it. On the weekend he'd put it out the driveway and sell it. I never thought about that until right this minute but I sort of carried on that tradition, you know? Anyway, he loved it. He had retail in his veins. He did. He liked it a lot, you know. You can say anything you want about faith or God or what you might think about. But somebody like my father to marry my mother because she was pregnant or whatever reason. Come into a situation where he was - ran the business which his father-in-law ran, you know. That's pretty kind of a rarity to have that situation, you know. Got to be something. Maybe it's just by accident. I just tell you that because . . . my father died of a gun shot wound to his head. Period.

I know two other folks who their father died of suicide. All three used the same tool – a gun! They might not have shot themselves in the head exactly. I tried to not get that specific with them but they all died. One of them went to the funeral home; shot himself in the car. Had the . . . had the residence all cleaned out; cleaned it all up so they could sell it. Planned. Came to the beach near here to take care of this lady because she was sick. Then he went back north. Did it like he had it . . . it was all ready to be done. There's a word I use when you have a child. When you're carrying . . . not a word. There's a saying I have - when you're carrying that child out of the hospital, they give you a stupid pill you have to take. Otherwise you can't take the child out of the hospital. At any rate he went to the funeral home. The other person I knew was a teenager. Found the body. I don't know where he did it but he did it on their property.

So there's got to be - call it what you want. I can't imagine, you know, my father finding his way to do it; and me encounter two other people who have the same situation. My mom seemed to handle her shock of it pretty good. You know, I . . . I'll just say this about myself. I was . . . I'm always, always been probably, always will be, worse when younger - I was pretty really self-absorbed. That's all I can say. I mean I was there. I lived it like she lived it. We had conversations about it. Yeah, we learned to pay the bills together because he paid the bills, you know. So we sat down and well, she had some idea, you know, you got the bills; not too complicated to write the check; slide it in the envelope. But none the less, a lot to learn in a hurry. Back then they gave you an envelope insert with your bill for whatever, and it was a prepaid postage tag. Thinking back I recall, he couldn't drive around. I know he had . . . I know he bought a . . . I don't know what he had but I know he had a car, you know, when he died. No note neither. Don't even know if I would have wanted one. Don't know about that. Just . . . it all hurts. It's all painful.

I can do a lot of asides. My . . . my mother and father . . . my father used to love dogs. They built this new house. My mother vowed they'd never be a dog in it. So after . . . after some years, maybe not very long, but after some point in time, my father found a place in Pulaski, New York which was selling poodles who weren't registered. They were just . . . they didn't shed. He took my mother up there. Got her to . . . got her to go along with buying this dog. At the end of my father's life, that dog was still alive. One of the things my mother mentioned to me, which I still think about, is the fact that he went down into that basement. He asked the dog to go with him. I believe my father would never have asked that dog to go with him if he was gonna shoot himself. I'm not saying he didn't go down there, maybe to think about trying it out. See how it might work or whatever, you know. But he wouldn't have invited that dog to go with him. Well, the dog did go. He loved him, the dog. I don't think he'd do that in front of the dog. I don't. You can look at it another way. Put it maybe he wanted the dog to warn somebody, too? Maybe the shot would warn so maybe . . . I don't know. He was able to do it on his own.

I have to live it that way. It's better for me. He coulda wanted company, too. I don't know. I don't know. I never thought about the wanting company part until I just said it. Doesn't matter. It's a lot of years ago. I coped by staying self-absorbed, in my world. I was doing well. I was on construction. Things were good for me. I was making a good dollar. I didn't have to kill myself because of time and materials - all that stuff, so I just . . . something else just popped into my brain. I was gonna tell you that, too, and I forgot what it was. Anyway . . .

Talking about all this, I can't help not think of what my dad would be thinking, were he still here, of me becoming a two millionaire. And it makes me want to cry. Can not hold back the tears even. I can't imagine what he'd say. His pride would be . . . he'd tell his neighbor. If he was still in Scriba, he'd be telling anybody that would listen to him. I don't know exactly but I'd have to stifle him. My experience has been, you know, I . . . was really high when I made my number. A friend tells me this about myself. The reason I don't have very many friends is because I set the standard too high. If my standard for friends is to take as good a care of me as my parents did, they will always fail the test. Nobody's gonna do that for me. I have one diploma from the Mullan/Davis/Leger family which has allowed me to live my entire life comfortably without a doubt. If it were not for them, there is no way I would be here in any way, shape or form. I would have been a walking disaster.

I shared that two number by the way with a few people here in this building. They in turn had shared it with somebody else. I wished I hadn't done that because doesn't anybody need to know what I got. I got what I got. That's what I got. If I was poor, I wouldn't be here. That's an obvious thing. I don't know what wealth is. Anytime I can live in a building where people come pay money to stay at a Resort where I live all year round, I figure I'm living pretty good, so to speak. Then again, since I had to do the math for you, I guess I was a pretty odd Drifter for 13 or so years. Just never noticed. Keeping it simple for me is my world.

Took me a year to work on this story. So I have to start to wrap it up with another story since it's now late May, 2019. Biden, did you know he's a Syracuse Law graduate?. Do you know that? I only lived there. As for the current President, a business man, let me make it clear first. I didn't vote for him. I think it's better. I think it's better. I think it will be better for the people of the United States. I think he likes the Country. He's got an odd ball personality. Doesn't come off real good when he says things and he definitely lies, you know, without question. But I think he has the Country at heart. And I wouldn't vote for him again either. Policy? There's hope. Personality? Deranged about describes it.

I could go on and on forever. One more story less serious than suicide or stocks. Because of my hobby as I call it, one of the stocks I owned early on, and I don't own it anymore, was Holiday Inn. In 1970 I took my first trip to Daytona with my mother and father of course. Drove down I-95. Wasn't finished in them days. You had to go through Georgia. You had to get off and ramble through it, but on I-95 there were Holiday Inns everywhere. They had a service which they offered you. You drove in. There was lunch; they had a buffet. They had a . . . I think they had breakfast in the morning even back then. And when you got up in the morning, they could calculate how far you were gonna be able to get the next day. You could make a reservation at the desk. Hit the road and then you could just drive right in there the next day. I thought this has got to be the greatest company that ever was. You know, they got to make a lot of money so I was back buying those ten shares back then or whatever I bought. I owned it for a long time.

Years go by. Mr. Trump! I never heard of him before. He went into a partnership as a franchisee in Atlantic City. I believe it was a casino hotel combined but I don't know what it was. It was at least a hotel. It was on the ocean front and it was Holiday Inn. And Trump was the franchise owner. That's a lot of years ago. This is what I remember. At some point in time Mr. Trump decided that Holiday Inn was not running the place correctly. He wanted them out. He's gonna sue them for the right to take it over. Apparently, they didn't give up easily. So it was front page news in New York State, all around the State, that somebody was challenging the Holiday Inn for rights to own it. You thought to yourself, this guy's got to be an idiot. He's going up against the Holiday Inn? Who could be any dumber than that? Well, he won! He took it over, put the Trump name on it.

So there's a guy in this building who I've told that story to. He's an avid Republican. He's the older night guy.

He says, "I retell that story often".

It's a true story. I can't tell you whether it was a casino or not. The moral of the story is that the man's so pushy, he gets what he wants. You know, if it costs whatever it costs, it costs. You know, it's a fact that his fortune has dissipated since he became President. It don't seem to be bothering him. It was bothering him, he'd say, "Okay, see you guys. Take over this thing", you know?

Stay tuned I guess.

I don't know a thing about any of the Russian attacks. What I know is what I've listened to and paid attention to is only what affects my life. I bought a little bit of Facebook and they got big troubles. I bought it a little while ago and I sold it. It's already gone. You know I never buy and sell that fast. I have a . . . there's a guy on one of the financial cable shows, has a theory. Don't quote me from my explanation. He says if you buy . . . if you think you're gonna . . . if you think you're not ready to get into a stock but you want to get into it, you buy 25% now. Then there's a number he used. I had to make up one for myself. After it goes up a certain percentage, then you buy another 25%. After it goes up, I haven't reached the other percentage yet, but after it goes up another percentage, you put the rest of it in – the other 50% say. So I bought several things on that premise where I put 25% in. I've sold a few of those already; they've gone down. I use the number . . . I don't like to lose more than 12% – 15%. I just don't like to lose that much. I have to keep it simple for myself. If it rises 20%; I don't make some calculation. Once it drops 12 – 15% anywhere on the scale, I get out. I don't have the . . . I don't have the ability. I can't figure out how to engineer that when it fluctuates up, then down and up again. Like certainly now, things have probably fluctuated down. You know what I mean? I call it my cushion. But it would be a good way to do that if you could program it.

So now I come to my last word. What I know about things for older people is, they don't have enough. I don't know how much enough is for each person, but they don't have enough. Now you know why you, and everyone, should be able to manage it so you have enough when the time comes. To manage it without . . . without . . . aw heck; I already told ya. If I'm comfortable being old, that's the only reason I'm comfortable being old - because I'm comfortable financially. That's, you know, I don't like being old but financially, I don't have nothin to worry about. If I lived to be a hundred, I still don't have nothin to worry about.

I never thought the following words would come out of my mouth: "I am really proud of myself". Telling you this story just blows me away. I never thought I would tell any one person about suicide or my dad's dark side or my mom's mistakes or my struggle to say thank you or my hobby. I am not an expert on anything but my own story, my own world and my own way of doin stuff. But I know something for sure now. When someone is feeling down, or in a life change or whatever, ASK them if they are thinking of hurting themselves. ASK them and get them to a professional NOW. You will feel better and you may save a life. That's the weird part we never know about when suicide doesn't happen – the part about whether like a gunshot wound to the head would have happened or not. Period.

You didn't used to know nothin about me, and now you know more than most of it. Now the whole world will know. It terrifies me and shrinks me even smaller to be safe in my shell.

THE END

ACKNOWLEDGEMENTS

I shall remain indebted to all these people as I roll out this series of profiles on "*Broken Giants*". Each awakened or encouraged or moved me to accept the mystery of the gift of expressing truth.

Glenn, a mentor and
brother for a lifetime
Kat and Shelley, my
west coast daughters
Kathleen and Dick, first
trusted their Cous
JJG, first recognized a dia-
mond in the rough
Deni, remains my pub-
lishing guardian angel
Al, yanked me to take a
step back and regroup
The Resort Staff, make
my life a dream daily
The Caffreys, so many
give so much
Bobbie, inhaled my art
to find its heart here

Linda, first connected
me to love in Parker
Eddie & Elisabeth, touch
me like no other
Monika and Helga, sus-
tained me back when
Dr. Mike, who befriended
me, alone, in Alaska
John & Mary, who ac-
cepted a rookie Therapist
Margaret, Sunil, Bill & TB
who taught me LTC
Nicole, whose silent tal-
ents absorb my voice
Tana & Teddy and
Taneyhill, lifelong Buds
Tom, our own gifted MSS
'62 Thomas Merton

Trudi, Quinn, Alena,
Blake and Chuck, my east
MI and east coast clan
Denis, modeled being a writer
so early in our careers
Hiedi, awakened my con-
fidence and strengths
Diane, lovingly ed-
ited and inspired
Marianne, added the artis-
tic connection to the cover
Alice at Ball State, first trusted
me to shake things up
Mike Mullan, chose to
risk expanding his life
long comfort zone
Bonnie, has supported

so long from so far
Nguyen Dang The, keeping me
safe all over II Corps, RVN
Steve & Diane, parented me
through Edelgard's death
Dorothy, being so level-
headed for 40 years
Frank & Joe & Mike, whose
own arts inspired me
Lynda, Gloria & Marge, al-
lowed me to be safe whenever
Barbara and Francie, modeled
gentle power and wisdom
Bill O', modeled how an MFT
Pro can just be who we are
Traci, a quiet example to me in
Denver of integrity of spirit

About the Author

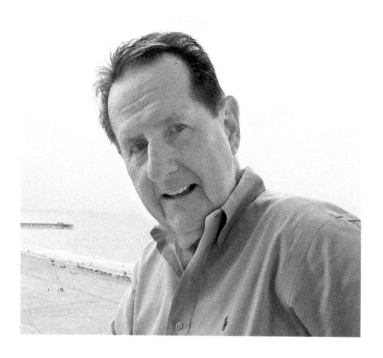

First time author & retired Marriage & Family Therapist Pat Clisham engaged theater arts early on as a student appearing in major roles; followed by producing and directing 4 popular full length plays in college theater; followed by the H C Curry role in "The Rainmaker" at the Pensacola Little Theater in 1973. Now by way of Viet Nam, Beirut, Iraq, Afghanistan and California in multiple high level occupations in Army Intelligence, business and mental health care, he shifts his focus to writing and residing in Myrtle Beach, SC.

Lightning Source UK Ltd.
Milton Keynes UK
UKHW041528191119
353829UK00001B/298/P